DRUG LAG

DRUG LAG

Federal Government Decision Making

RITA RICARDO CAMPBELL, Ph.D.
with a foreword by
WILLIAM M. WARDELL, M.D., Ph.D.

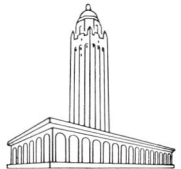

HOOVER INSTITUTION PRESS 1976
STANFORD, CALIFORNIA 94305

Acknowledgments

I wish to thank especially Dr. William Wardell, who has been my informal tutor in the field of pharmacology, and also my associate Gerald Musgrave, Ph.D.

The Hoover Institution on War, Revolution and Peace, founded at Stanford University in 1919 by the late President Herbert Hoover, is a center for advanced study and research on public and international affairs in the twentieth century. The views expressed in its publications are entirely those of the authors and do not necessarily reflect the views of the staff, officers, or Board of Overseers of the Hoover Institution.

Hoover Institution Studies 55

© 1976 by the Board of Trustees of the
    Leland Stanford Junior University
All rights reserved
International Standard Book Number: 0-8179-3552-5
Library of Congress Catalog Card Number: 76-26772
Printed in the United States of America

Contents

Foreword	vii
Introduction	1
The National Advisory Drug Committee (NADC)	3
Evolution of Drug Efficacy Criteria	5
Risk-Benefit and Cost-Benefit	6
NADC's Early Involvement	7
Drug Lag Issues	14
Role of the Economist	20
A New FDA Commissioner	24
FDA Considers Cost-Benefit Analysis	27
Pressures on FDA	29
FDA's Position on Drug Lag Changes	34
What Was the Role of Cost-Benefit Analysis in the Drug Lag Issue?	38
The Public Interest	42
Selected Bibliography	55

Foreword

This book is important for several reasons. It is a valuable historical document of the activities of a major FDA outside advisory committee—the National Advisory Drug Committee—and the way this committee was used by FDA to handle and formulate a response to a major scientific and public policy issue, the "drug lag." As a founder member of this committee, Dr. Rita Ricardo Campbell was privy to many meetings and policy discussions, of which those of us involved in the scientific debate outside the FDA were only dimly aware. Her careful chronological documentation (including, for example, comparisons of the information available to FDA with that actually supplied to the committee) gives pause to those of us who believe in the value of outside advisory committees, and inevitably raises the question: how can an advisory committee be truly independent?

Students of political science and government policymaking in general (particularly the crucial science-public policy interface), as well as those interested in the behind-the-scenes regulatory politics of the drug lag issue, will find this a fascinating account and a valuable addition to the slender resource material available on this subject.

This book is also valuable as a professional economist's view of how cost-benefit analyses can and should contribute to the quality of decision making at the science-public policy interface. Again there is a useful historical analysis of how this issue arose to become part of FDA's decision making. This aspect of the process is still only in its infancy; students of this topic would be well advised to start with this account as they follow developments in the future.

William Wardell, M.D., Ph.D.
Associate Professor of Pharmacology, Toxicology, and of Medicine
Director, Center for the Study of Drug Development
University of Rochester, New York

DRUG LAG:
FEDERAL GOVERNMENT
DECISION MAKING*

Introduction

Some academic economists believe that decision making by federal government employees at the higher grades is based primarily on cost-benefit analysis or economic criteria rather than on the major political criterion of how many votes the decision will gain or lose. It is generally accepted that elected federal officials view a public policy problem primarily in terms of political gains or losses, rather than to assess economic benefits and costs of a range of options. In some cases the preferred political and economic solutions may be the same. When they are not in agreement, it is accepted under the theory of democratic government that political judgment takes precedence. However, as government regulations expand into the complex areas of basic and applied research and technology, pressure develops for decisions that can be logically defended by use of scientifically acceptable data.

Appointed government officials are also subject to political pressures since they must testify before congressional subcommittees and also annually justify the amount of dollars which they feel Congress should appropriate. Therefore, they also may tend to make decisions more on a political than on an economic basis.

Whether federal employees in the upper grades, who come up through the system and may or may not be filling a job at the political appointee level, also place a greater weight on political rather than economic criteria, is a question that appears to be debatable. Although during recent years the economists' technique of cost-benefit analysis has become more acceptable in Washing-

---

*Revision and expansion of paper given at the Western Economic Association's annual meeting in San Francisco, June 26, 1976.

ton, D.C., documentation of specific decisions based on this approach indeed seems difficult to find.

A cost-benefit analysis sums up all the data, both the benefits and the costs, which can be measured by a single unit—dollars—in order to obtain a net benefit or loss for a particular proposed policy. It is recognized that not all information is always available, nor can all information which is available be always measured by dollars; but to the extent that the latter is possible it is advisable to do so and then to list those items, both costs and benefits, which are not included in the univariate measure, the dollar. The policymaker should be presented the cost-benefit analysis with *caveats* as to what is omitted, any assumptions made, and how each policy decision may redistribute income. Executive Order 11821, effective in spring 1975, has forced all federal government agencies to use this type of analysis to determine whether their proposed regulations might have an inflationary impact on the economy.

In 1974, I participated in a National Academy of Sciences workshop on "Decision Making for Regulating Chemicals in the Environment" and was involved specifically in the group which wrote the chapter "Information on Benefits," which is the concluding chapter of that printed report. It states as follows:

> Economic costs and benefits are likely to be basic considerations in regulatory decisions. Thus it is important that an appropriate conceptual framework be used to define and, where possible, to measure economic costs and benefits. When regulatory decisions are expected to cause changes in the output of goods and services, the net economic value of these changes should be measured in dollar terms, using the principles of willingness to pay and opportunity cost, and they should be included in the information presented to the decision maker. . . .
>
> There is no fully objective way of arraying such information. But the costs and benefits can be measured approximately, and the resulting information can be aggregated into a sufficiently small number of elements that a decision maker can grasp the potential effects of a decision and can comprehend the differences in effect produced by alternate choices.[1]

A recent example in which cost-benefit analysis appears to have been used and which resulted in a Food and Drug Administration (FDA) regulation, May 9, 1975, was the drug lag issue. In this matter an advisory committee to

---

1. *Decision Making for Regulating Chemicals in the Environment* (Washington, D.C.: National Academy of Sciences, 1975), pp. 62-63.

the FDA, the National Advisory Drug Committee (NADC), rather than government staff members, played a major role in bringing about greater use of a cost-benefit approach. The appointment in 1973 of a new FDA commissioner, Alexander Schmidt, M.D., and the development of a Washington, D.C. climate more favorable towards cost-benefit analysis were also major factors.

The National Advisory Drug Committee (NADC)

The Food and Drug Administration (FDA) is a scientific regulatory Agency responsible for the safety of the Nation's foods, cosmetics, drugs, medical devices, biologics, and electronic radiological products.

The manufacturer has the prime responsibility for assuring the safety of its products. FDA's role is to monitor the industry and to provide the consumer the best assurances possible that the industry is meeting its responsibility.[2]

Commissioner Edwards, M.D., during the first meeting of the National Advisory Drug Committee, gave the following "charge" to the committee:

To advise and consult with the Secretary or his designee on policies, programs, and planning for marshalling necessary resources to meet broad major problems and responsibilities in drug related programs of the Food and Drug Administration.

The Committee will review and evaluate Agency programs and provide advice and guidance to the Secretary or his designee on policy matters of national significance relating to FDA's statutory mission in the area of drugs.

The Committee will provide advice and recommendations on such issues of national concern as over-the-counter drugs, oral contraceptives, adverse drug reaction monitoring systems, and revision of New Drug Application review procedures.

It will serve as a forum for the exchange of views and recommendations not otherwise available to FDA on program direction and effectiveness.[3]

Most of the NADC members had expertise in a professional field. Among them were three practicing physicians: a pediatrician specializing in allergies, a psychiatrist, and a surgeon; as well as the medical director of the Ochsner Clinic. Academic representatives included a dean of a school of nursing, a

---

2. U.S. HEW, FDA, *FY 1976 PMS Blue Book,* April 1975, p. 9.
3. U.S. FDA, NADC *Minutes of the First Meeting,* April 20, 1972, p. 5.

dean of a school of medicine, a dean of a college of pharmacy, a director of pharmaceutical services in a southern university, a professor of biostatistics, a professor of electrical engineering, and myself, an economist. Additionally, there was a physician, who was president and chief executive officer of a large pharmaceutical company, a pharmacist, a president and director of a small medical devices firm, a former social worker, a "specialist" in the New York investment market, and a "consumer." The limit was eighteen members; another academician, an anesthesiologist, was added to make this total. Individuals were rotated off in groups of three, starting as early as April 1973, a year after the first meeting, but only six months after the initial presentation of the drug lag issue to the committee.[4]

In March 1975, the three top public advisory committees which report directly to the Commissioner of the FDA (on Drugs, Food, and Veterinary Medicine) were merged and nine members of the NADC were made members of the newly merged National Advisory Food and Drug Committee (NAFDC), which met for the first time at the end of March 1975. By October 1975, only five of the original NADC members were still on that committee. These three original, general, public advisory committees which merged to form the NAFDC were composed of outside consultants with a much broader representation of expertise than the usual, more limited, scientific outside advisory committees to the FDA. For example, the members of the Cardiovascular and Renal Advisory Committee ". . . are selected from leaders in the field of cardiovascular and renal disorders and related medical and scientific disciplines" and their function is to advise "the Commissioner regarding the safety and efficacy of drugs employed in the field of cardiovascular and renal disorders and the advances, changing concepts, and trends in the therapy of these disorders."[5]

As of April 1974 and April 1975, only the Veterinary Medicine Committee had a lawyer, and I was the only economist on these three "top level" advisory committees and subsequently the merged committee.[6]

On September 28, 1972, the first day of the third meeting of FDA's National Advisory Drug Committee (which was the first meeting of that committee which I attended as a member), Henry Simmons, M.D., then Director of FDA's Bureau of Drugs, gave a lengthy presentation listed on the agenda as

---

4. The first meeting was primarily a briefing of the members and the second meeting was a one-day meeting, called on less than twenty-four hours notice to consider a ban on DES in cattle feed.
5. U.S. FDA, *Public Advisory Committees: Authority, Structure, Functions, Members,* April 1974, p. 36.
6. Ibid., pp. 5, 7, 9; and April 1975 edition, pp. 5, 7.

"Effects of the 1962 Amendments on Drug Research and Development."[7] The presentation was intended to be a partial answer to charges by academic medical researchers that (a) FDA had failed to approve therapeutically beneficial drugs which were available abroad and (b) therefore, that the United States was experiencing a drug lag especially as compared to Great Britain.

Evolution of Drug Efficacy Criteria

The basic 1938 Drug Act required that FDA evaluate the safety of new drugs, but did not require (although it did permit) the evaluation of efficacy. In 1962, the law was amended to require FDA to assess also the efficacy of all drugs both new and old. This was partly an emotional response by Congress to the "thalidomide tragedy" of severely deformed infants born to mothers who had taken the German tranquilizing drug thalidomide, introduced in 1958, and withdrawn internationally in November 1961. Neither France nor the United States had approved the drug. The United States, under its then existing law requiring proof of safety, had several times rejected approval at the end of each sixty-day application period on the grounds that data of proof of safety were inadequate.[8] The incident made a heroine of Dr. Frances Kelsey and assured passage of the 1962 amendments. Generally overlooked, however, were the facts that the existing law did protect persons in the United States; that laboratory tests of the effects of thalidomide on pregnant mice, rats and other common laboratory animals, with the exception of a few species of rabbits, could not detect fetal deformities; and that the new efficacy requirement, although passed in response to the thalidomide problem, would not directly protect against another similar incident.

The FDA evaluates applications for clinical investigation of new drugs (INDs) and for marketing new drugs (NDAs) in the United States. It does this with in-house personnel. To judge the efficacy of a drug, as well as its safety, FDA was forced to develop criteria of the "substantial evidence" section of the 1962 law which are acceptable to the scientific community. These criteria were finally published as regulations on May 8, 1970, although efficacy criteria had been implemented much earlier by many companies. The preferred evidence is

---

7. Among other FDA staff present were the Commissioner Charles Edwards, M.D.; Mark Novitch, M.D., Deputy Associate Commissioner for Medical Affairs; Marion Finkel, M.D., Deputy Director, Bureau of Drugs; and Richard Crout, M.D., Director, Office of Scientific Evaluation, Bureau of Drugs.

8. Some observers believe that simple procrastination is more like the truth.

from the controlled double-blind, clinical study in which neither the physician nor the patient knows who receives the drug being tested and who receives the control drug, usually a placebo. In 1972, most of FDA's staff working on prescription drugs were physicians and scientists who had little or no knowledge of economic cost-benefit analysis, but were familiar with the implicit types of risk-benefit analysis that characterize biological and medical decisions.

Risk-Benefit and Cost-Benefit

The use of the term "risk-benefit" rather than "cost-benefit" seems to equate biological "risks" with all the "costs" incurred and to define "benefits" as only "good" benefits uncorrected for any negative benefits or losses. Thus society's costs are underestimated in "risk-benefit" decisions.[9]

The costs of society in loss of potential benefits from a drug not allowed to be marketed are often overlooked; for example, when the biological risk of serious effects to the user is considered to be high and the disease for which the drug is taken is not a terminal one. If the disease is terminal, as for example many types of cancer are, then approval to market a drug which appears to be more efficacious than drugs already on the market is likely to be given well before all the data on probable adverse side effects are known.

The uncertainty of a low probability of a serious side effect of an otherwise beneficial drug without an equally efficacious substitute may remain unknown over a great number of years. The rarer the disease and/or the side effect, the more likely that this would be the case. If the risk is only one in 500,000, it could take 500,000 persons exposed for that side effect to appear. Meanwhile if the drug is not approved and the disease is terminal, thousands of deaths would needlessly occur while waiting for evidence of the rare side effect. If the disease is serious but not terminal, thousands of persons would needlessly suffer.

The estimates of what degree of biological risk may be acceptable for some degree of benefit are subjective value judgments and are generally not based on hard data. Moreover:

The expert is inclined to believe that people of his own professional background are more likely to make responsible and defensible judgments than are non-experts. The non-experts may, on the other hand, be suspicious of the expert as biased or parochial. Moreover, the idea that

---

9. Rita R. Campbell, *Food Safety Regulation* (Washington, D.C.: AEI, August 1974), p. 19.

experts agree is usually a myth. There are many situations in which one can get respected experts to disagree quite vigorously, as testified by the textbook *Controversy in Internal Medicine* . . . .[10]

Experts often disagree because data are incomplete and the issues are very complex.

A difficulty in weighing large risks, sometimes of unknown probability, to a few persons against relatively small benefits to many people is that the significance of the large risk and its possible horror to the individual are more easily comprehended and thus well publicized. On the other hand, the relatively small benefit to each individual has little public impact, even though when multiplied manifold it may become much larger in total. Thus even the existence of these benefits, actual and potential, is often unknown by the person who may benefit. It is natural that those who make the law and those who administer it are far more likely to emphasize a large risk to an individual, even though it be of very rare incidence, rather than the possibility of a high total of net social benefits accruing to many persons minus the costs of the risks incurred. . . . In addition, the individual's risk or cost is a private cost which can sometimes be insured against. Thus there is the possibility of recovering money through civil law action. The loss sustained by never receiving a benefit is a social, noninsurable cost against which there is no legal recovery. It is a matter of degree and therefore of judgment to decide what fraction, if any, of high risk to an individual is acceptable as a tradeoff for sizable total benefits to many. "Is it to be one in a million, or lower, or higher?"[11]

NADC's Early Involvement

A letter dated February 29, 1972, signed by Robert Dripps, M.D., of the University of Pennsylvania Medical School and by twenty other medical researchers, including Nobel Prize winner Dr. Dickinson Richards, Dr. Michael deBakey, and others of similar stature, was presented to the National Advisory Drug Committee on the morning of September 28, 1972. The letter charged that " . . . the procedures by which new drugs are evaluated and approved for use in this country is [*sic*] causing us to fall behind in this important area of medical science"—or in other words that the United States was experiencing vis-à-vis other countries a drug lag because ". . .the

---

10. William Wardell and Louis Lasagna, *Regulation of Drug Development* (Washington, D.C.: AEI, 1975), p. 38. Refers to *Controversy in Internal Medicine,* vol. 1, edited by F.J. Ingelfinger, A.S. Relman, and M. Finland (Philadelphia: Saunders, 1966). See also *Controversy in Internal Medicine,* vol. 2, edited by Ingelfinger et al. (Philadelphia: Saunders, 1974).

11. Campbell, op. cit., pp. 22-23.

regulatory system . . . too often stifles creativity and escalates costs of research."[12] A second letter, dated March 22, 1972, which contained back-up data, stated that " . . . we do know there are increasing signs that drug development in this country is lagging." This letter was distributed to the NADC the afternoon of September 28, in response to committee request.[13] It had been placed on the meeting table in front of the members of the NADC while they ate luncheon together downstairs, apart from FDA officials and staff. Only at the end of that afternoon did the discussion return to the Dripps Committee letters. The NADC transcript of the next day's meeting indicates that many, and possibly all, Committee members had not received the full letter.

> Dr. Campbell: I don't know whether I got a defective copy, but I never got the last page of the second letter, so I still don't know who signed it or how it actually ended. All I have is the first three pages.
>
> Dr. Moxley: That is all we all got. . . .
>
> Dr. Edwards: Why didn't they get the last page of the second letter? Let's give it to them. We will get that for you before you leave.[14]

The Dripps letter of March 22, 1972, was seven pages long and went far beyond the drug lag issue, but much of the additional material in the latter pages of the letter was relevant.

Twenty-one persons signed the first Dripps Committee letter of February 29, 1972; Dr. Dripps alone signed the second and third letters of March 22 and August 4, 1972, respectively; but twenty-one persons signed the fourth letter of September 24, 1973; and twenty-two persons were identified as members of the "Ad Hoc Committee . . . of the medical and scientific community" in the Dripps statement of November 30, 1972.

The first two letters were addressed to Congressman Paul Rogers and not to the commissioner of FDA. This created a defensive, justification posture rather than an investigative one by FDA.

---

12. Letter to the Honorable Paul Rogers, House of Representatives, mimeo, p. 1.
13. Committee members commented as follows:
Mr. Middleton: "Some of us had not received the second letter. . . ." Dr. Mark Novitch: "I think it [the second letter] was signed by Dripps on behalf of the committee. . .a lot of them refused to take any responsibility for the second letter which contained assertions that I thought were a little further out than the first ones. So that they take full responsibility for the first letter, but only indirect and very partial responsibility for the second letter." Dr. Edwards: "I still think as Jack [Moxley] pointed out, however, their names are on it." NADC *Transcript,* September 29, 1972, p. 55.
14. Ibid. The author's copy of the second Dripps letter has only Dr. Dripp's signature, which is in contradiction to Dr. Edward's remark cited in footnote 13.

Later in testimony, Dr. Simmons argued that there was a worldwide decline in discovery of new drugs which was not unique to the United States. Moreover, the decline had started in the United States earlier than 1962 (the date of the amendments) and, therefore, a drug lag in market availability of new effective drugs in the United States vis-à-vis other countries did not exist.

The *Summary Minutes* of the NADC September meeting do not reflect fully some of the members' pronounced skepticism towards FDA's case that ". . .the experts who signed a [sic] letter were criticizing a system that did not exist today. . . . This was a system where a closed FDA made its judgments in isolation and let nobody else look at the data or enter into that decision making with them."[15] According to the transcript, Dr. Edwards stated: "I think I in no way question the integrity of any of the members that signed it. I think they were misled and given poor advice by—as I said, I think it was an outside organization—and I think they were naive."[16] Further, after much discussion, Dr. Moxley, then Dean, School of Medicine, University of Maryland, stated, "I can't believe that this group of men have nothing but innuendo to back up their case."[17] Dr. Youngue, a practicing psychiatrist, added, "I feel pretty much the same way."[18] Other members commented in a similar fashion, and Dr. Edwards remarked on the following morning that: "You also obviously felt that the charges that were made by the Dripps Committee are important enough that they certainly ought to be answered. . . ."[19]

The commissioner asked the NADC to make a formal statement on the charge of drug lag. However, the committee refused at that September meeting to state a position on drug lag but rather approved the following "Summary Statement" on September 29, 1972:

> As a closing action of the third meeting of the National Advisory Drug Committee, this council has moved to issue a joint statement, summarizing its conclusions from this conference and recommending a course of action to be pursued by its membership.
>
> 1. Based on the presentation of the Bureau of Drugs at this meeting, the preliminary impression of this Committee is that the Agency has established an effective scientific method for the review of New Drug Applications. The reviews and evaluations as accomplished in

---

15. Henry Simmons in NADC *Summary Minutes,* September 28, 1972, p. 5.
16. NADC *Transcript,* September 28, 1972, p. 50.
17. Ibid., p. 87.
18. Ibid.
19. NADC *Transcript,* September 29, 1972, pp. 3, 4.

the Bureau of Drugs would appear to fulfill the legislative requirements governing the safety and efficacy of therapeutic products.

2. The Committee, however, is requesting the Bureau of Drugs to provide a further detailed presentation with specific data covering the following activities:
    a. Implementation of voluntary compliance.
    b. The effectiveness of the labeling of therapeutic products.

3. Having read the correspondence from the Dripps Committee and reviewed the allegations thereof, the initial conclusion of the Committee is that further substance would have to be presented by that group to substantiate its charges. For this reason, the National Advisory Drug Committee is requesting that Dr. Dripps or his representative present their position directly to the National Advisory Drug Committee.

4. To insure that the Committee has received a comprehensive presentation of the opposing positions relating to drug approvals, the Committee is also requesting that representatives from each of the following groups be invited to present their arguments at the next meeting of the National Advisory Drug Committee:
    a. Industry
    b. Congress
    c. Consumer

This meeting is to be scheduled in November, 1972.

No mention was made by FDA of an August 4, 1972, letter by Dr. Dripps to Secretary Edwards which covered several points raised during the June 6 meeting, including:

> Should not the data base on which we are operating be updated and expanded so that all of us have a better perspective on where we are going in drug research in this country? Some examples might be:
>
> a) An analysis of INDs and NDAs on a case-by-case basis, not only from the point of view of FDA but the investigator and sponsor, as well. This would pinpoint and identify causes for delay. (p.2)

And the letter concluded:

> ...we believe and hope FDA's leadership will support the proposal of our committee, namely, that Congressman Paul Rogers' Subcommittee on Public Health and Environment establish an expert advisory committee to study and review the effect of the 1962 Drug Act and Regulations on the practice of medicine and the conduct of academic and industrial drug research. An information base built on reliable data

will help insure that the Congress, as it considers changes in the drug regulatory system, will do so in a manner which fosters research and the development of new safe and effective drug products. (pp.2, 3)

Dr. Dripps, accompanied by Dr. Louis Lasagna and others representing different points of view also spoke on November 30, 1972, at the NADC meeting.[20] A logical explanation given for addressing the earlier letters of the Dripps *ad hoc* committee to Congressman Paul Rogers rather than to FDA officials was that the U.S. House of Representatives Subcommittee on Public Health and Environment "has funds and the authority to commission an outside study by experts" and this the Dripps Committee thought was desirable.[21] In his presentation, Dr. Dripps expressed dismay that even after their apparently friendly meeting of June 6 with FDA's top officials to streamline procedural processing of INDs and NDAs, FDA's attitude remained as implied during the September NADC meeting, "that its [Dripps Committee] members were naive and had been misled."

Dr. Dripps stated:

> At our meeting on June 6, we heard from Dr. Simmons substantially what he told you at your meeting in September. His main point was that the decline in the discovery and introduction of new drugs is a worldwide phenomenon, not restricted to the United States. Data on which this view was based were developd by the West German pharmaceutical manufacturer, Boehringer Sohn, of Ingelheim. . . . This study showed the decline in new drugs introduced to be more marked in this country than in others. If you will examine the table and chart at the end of my statement, which were derived from the Boehringer figures, you will see the decline in new drug introductions in the United States, from 31 in 1961 to five in 1970, more than accounts numerically for the worldwide decline of 22. Fifty-one new drugs were introduced elsewhere than in this country in 1961, and 55 in 1970. Does not this restatement of the Boehringer data suggest a new drug lag in our country, compared with the rest of the world?

And further:

> In Dr. Richard Crout's thought-provoking presentation on the work of FDA's Office of Scientific Evaluations, we learned that Office is handling a total pool of about 3,200 Investigational New Drug Applications and that an estimated 100 to 220 in the total pool may be

---

20. Speakers included Joseph Stetler, President of the Pharmaceutical Manufacturers' Association; Benjamin Gordon, staff, U.S. Select Committee on Small Business; and James Turner, a lawyer, formerly with Ralph Nader. A statement by Anita Johnson and Sidney Wolfe, M.D., representing Ralph Nader's Health Research Group was submitted.
21. Robert Dripps, Testimony before the NADC, November 30, 1972, mimeo, p. 2.

potentially important new therapies. Why, then, we wonder, do only three to five medically important new drugs clear the NDA process in a given year? . . . (p. 8)

> The future of U.S. leadership in chemotherapeutpcs may be wrapped up in the answers to the subtle and complex question of why there are "drop-outs." We need to know how the criteria for performing and interpreting animal and human studies is [sic] affecting the fruits of therapeutic research. Is the risk-to-benefit equation set at a proper level to prevent the premature discard of potentially valuable drugs? The present system is inherently designed to err on the safe side. We urge a complete and thorough study of individual case histories. This might help us better judge whether valuable compounds are being lost to men. . . . (pp. 8, 9)

Near the end of the statement the following question was asked:

> Is the FDA judge, jury and the prosecutor under the law or the regulations? (p. 9)

The NADC members were never officially informed by FDA of many significant concurrent developments, both in FDA and outside, on the drug lag issue. For example, on June 6, 1972, FDA's commissioner and top staff had met with six members of the Dripps Committee.[22] Mention of that meeting, but not of the discussions which took place, was made by Dr. Edwards only in response to a question at the end of the morning session of the September 28, 1972, meeting. The relevant section of the transcript follows:

> Ms. Burnham: I was just going to ask, Dr. Edwards or Dr. Simmons, have any of you talked to any of the members of this Dripps Committee or only Dr. Dripps?
>
> Dr. Edwards: Came with two or three—how many were there, four or five—five of them. I have talked to a number of them individually, yes.
>
> Ms. Burnham: And they were aware of everything that was in the letter?
>
> Dr. Edwards: I would rather not speak for them. Several of them signed the letter having no idea of what was going to happen to the letter. As I say, I repeat for the fifth time today that I think, without going into any more detail, they were given damned poor advice. Any other comments?[23]

No mention was made by FDA of the letter of August 4, 1972, to Dr. Edwards which was a follow-up of the June 6 meeting at which it was agreed

---

22. *FDC Reports,* "The Pink Sheets," June 12, 1972, pp. 17, 18.
23. NADC *Transcript,* September 28, 1972, pp. 90, 91.

to have an interchange of questions. The existence of a fourth letter from the same Dripps Committee, dated September 24, 1973, was not revealed to members of the NADC until their meeting of July 18, 1974.

No mention was made during the NADC meetings of September 28-29, 1972—and then only a casual reference by FDA on November 30, 1972—of the detailed presentation by William Wardell, M.D., Ph.D., on "The Drug Lag: An International Comparison" read to the Fifth International Pharmacological Conference, July 1972. Dr. Richard Crout of FDA was present at the latter meeting and spoke against the points raised by Dr. Wardell. Dr. Lasagna referred during the November 30, 1972, NADC meeting to Dr. Wardell's survey data on

> . . . what competent clinicians in the United Kingdom think about the drugs they use (trying to hide from them which drugs we don't have so as not to bias their responses). As criticizable as these data may be, they are the best we have been able to come up with to give the reader an idea of what the United States patient might be losing out on by not having some of these drugs available. It's a tricky area because the research techniques are not generally available for trying to quantify what we are losing and what we are gaining by having a stricter form of control but we would be glad to supply the preliminary drafts of these two longish articles.
>
> Dr. Edwards: Dr. Wardell has sent me that through Dr. Campbell. I have specifically skirted the issue because it was a preliminary draft.
>
> Dr. Lasagna: You have seen the first of three articles and the second one is just about finished. I'm sure he will be glad to supply the other two. . . .[24]

There was during this period considerable turnover among the top staff of FDA, including the appointment of the new commissioner, Dr. Schmidt, and the replacement of Dr. Simmons, Director of the Bureau of Drugs, by the promotion of Dr. Richard Crout. These changes, and also bureaucratic inefficiencies, may explain why FDA made no attempt to keep committee members fully informed about actions of FDA in response to the charge of a drug lag. Commissioner Edwards had clearly thought ". . . that the instigation of the Dripps letter came from industry . . . [and a] particular company [was] involved. . . ."[25]

Commissioner Edwards stated early in the morning discussion of September 29, 1972, that it was his impression that there had been some misunder-

---

24. An unofficial transcript from a non-professional tape recording which has not been seen, reviewed, or discussed by those quoted, pp. 20, 21.
25. NADC *Transcript,* September 29, 1972, pp. 57, 58.

standing as to who was the chairman of the NADC. Dr. Simmons had stated earlier that he thought that John Moxley, M.D., who was a medical school dean, was the chairman,[26] but Edwards stated that he, the commissioner, ". . . was the chairman, and while there could conceivably be a change in the future, he thought that for the moment, while the Committee was still going through an organizational period, that it would be best to keep the chairmanship in his office."[27] The importance of who is chairman and who controls the agenda, as these factors influence decision outcomes, was clearly understood by Commissioner Edwards and subsequently by Commissioner Schmidt. At no time were the meetings chaired by other than the FDA commissioner or by top FDA staff.

Drug Lag Issues

Consideration of the drug lag was a major initial charge to the National Advisory Drug Committee. The issue was complex. There were and are differences of opinion in defining what is a *significant* new drug. The reliability of extrapolation of a drug's effects from experimental animals to humans is questionable.[28] Reliable data on the effect of new drugs on humans are scarce.

The statistical outcome of some prospective double-blind clinical studies is unreliable, as, for example, when the sample is initially too small or when too few persons remain in subsets because of a high refusal and/or drop-out rate. An unwise selection of a population at risk from which the matched controls may be chosen, substantial differences in the degree of illness of patients at the baseline, and the failure to rule out other independent variables at the baseline are other faults which occur sometimes in clinical drug studies. The effects of placebos and drugs may be obscured because of the difficulty in separating these effects from the natural course of healing of a disease. Errors in observations or even in transmission of records, and the patients' unreported and/or unobserved noncompliance in taking a prescribed drug or placebo, may cloud the conclusions. Thus the results of prospective short-run studies on the same drug do not always agree. Many studies which are retrospective either have methodological problems or involve too small a sample to make their value equal to prospective studies.

---

26. NADC *Transcript,* September 28, 1972, p. 169.
27. NADC *Summary Minutes,* September 29, 1972, p. 13.
28. See especially William Wardell, "Fluroxene and the Penicillin Lesson," *Anesthesiology,* vol. 38, no. 4, April 1973, pp. 309-12.

Furthermore, a negative trial can only conclude that no difference was demonstrated, not that there is no difference. The null hypothesis cannot be proved. Yet it is common to consider a negative trial as important evidence against the drug—perhaps more important than positive evidence. In fact, it should be just the other way around. Several well done positive trials by responsible investigators should be taken as evidence of efficacy, even in the face of a few negative trials, although a large number of the latter would obviously make one wonder about the general utility of the drug or the way in which it was being studied.[29]

Even more scarce are reliable data on the long-term effects of drugs on humans. The long-term effects of drugs which are not therapeutic for cancer but which might cause cancer are generally unknown and will remain so for many years until the scientific studies now underway, such as in-house studies at the National Center for Toxicological Research in Jefferson, Arkansas, or other long-run studies by academic and company researchers, are completed. Dr. C. Gordon Zubrod, Director of the Cancer Institute's activities in cancer treatment, states that, ". . . the lag period between the time a man is exposed to a chemical carcinogen and the time he develops cancer we know may be 10 to 30 years. . . ."[30]

Although all scientific data about benefits and costs are not usually available for a decision, the law requires that FDA make decisions to protect the consumer from unsafe and ineffective drugs. To delay a decision for any length of time is a decision—one which supports the *status quo*. The NADC members were repeatedly advised that if a drug company did not seek NDAs or did not wish to supply experimental drugs to U.S. physicians under INDs, then there was nothing FDA could do to make a drug which was developed abroad become available in the United States. The law gave a negative, not a positive mandate. This interpretation gradually has changed so that recently new guidelines for accepting research data on drugs developed abroad were announced in an FDA press release (April 8, 1975), as follows:

> . . . to encourage a freer flow of drug research information into the United States, reduce unnecessary duplication of such research, and thus speed FDA evaluation and public availability of significant new drugs that may be developed abroad.

Legal protection of company data because of trade secrets limits definitive analysis (even though more information would still be needed) of why some

---

29. Wardell and Lasagna, *Regulation and Drug Development,* p. 29.
30. C. G. Zubrod, testimony in U.S. Senate, Select Committee on Small Business, Subcommittee on Monopoly, in *Hearings on Competitive Problems in the Drug Industry,* 1973, part 23, p. 9674.

U.S. firms conduct research abroad and market abroad a significant new drug years ahead of marketing the same drug in the United States. Also hindered is analysis of the factors which make one drug company rather than another more successful in the development of significant new drugs.

Professor Peltzman's book, entitled *Regulation of Pharmaceutical Innovation*, is summarized as follows:

> ... the 1962 ("proof of efficacy") amendments ... (1) have cut the number of new drugs ... brought to the market each year by half with no corresponding reduction in inefficacious drugs, (2) have doubled the costs of drug development, (3) have increased drug prices by reducing competition among drugs (so that the sick pay $50 million more each year for drugs), and (4) have imposed substantial net social costs from deaths and illnesses that could have been prevented if the development of new drugs had not been hampered by the amendments.

Professor Peltzman also states that,

> the important conclusions of this study are that, perhaps before and certainly after 1962, too many resources have been devoted to testing of drug safety and efficacy before marketing and that, unless the law requiring proof of efficacy is rescinded, continued resource waste is inevitable. A favorable change in FDA procedures could reduce, but could never eliminate, the waste commanded by the law.[31]

In October 1972, I had received the preliminary draft copy of the article by Dr. William Wardell, University of Rochester Medical Center, "The Drug Lag: An International Comparison." This article was the first of three articles which were an expansion of his July 1972 paper given at the International Pharmacological Association meeting mentioned earlier. All three articles were published in *Clinical Pharmacology and Therapeutics* in 1973 and 1974.[32] The first article documents with data the classes of therapeutic drugs where a drug lag did exist in the United States as compared to Great Britain, which has a somewhat less restrictive policy governing approval of marketing of new drugs.

The first of Dr. Wardell's articles found that from 1962 to 1971 nearly four times as many new drugs became available in Great Britain as in the United States, and that for drugs marketed in both countries, about twice as many

---

31. Sam Peltzman, *Regulation of Pharmaceutical Innovation* (Washington, D.C.: AEI, 1974), back cover and p. 83. A popularized version of his earlier "The Benefits and Costs of New Drug Regulation" in *Regulating New Drugs,* edited by Richard Landau (Chicago: University of Chicago Press, 1973), which the author saw in draft form in late October 1972.

32. *Clinical Pharmacology and Therapeutics,* vol. 14, 1973, and vol. 15, 1974.

were introduced first in Great Britain as were introduced first in the United States. By therapeutic category, the drug lag was most marked in cardiovascular, gastrointestinal, respiratory, diuretic, and antibacterial drugs. His second article documents that specialist physicians at an American university medical center (Rochester) had a very low level of knowledge of new effective drugs available abroad but not in the United States; but when they did know of such drugs, usually they wished to have them available.

Wardell's third article, "Therapeutic Implications of the Drug Lag," which I received much later, can be summarized in part, as follows: On balance, Great Britain appears to have gained, in comparison with the United States, from its more permissive policy toward the marketing of new drugs coupled with a more rigorous program of post-marketing surveillance. Wardell would, therefore, intensify surveillance of new drugs *after* marketing in the United States.

Thus, supported by Professor Peltzman's econometric analysis of the issue, and especially by pharmacological information from Professor Wardell (a physician trained in clinical pharmacology and research techniques), I was able to analyze the statistical data and also name, during NADC meetings, effective therapeutic drugs which were then not available in the United States and for which no U.S. therapeutically equivalent substitute drugs existed. Without Wardell's data, Peltzman's study would have languished without any effect on national policy, as do many other excellent econometric studies, because of too rigid assumptions, reliance on equations for communication, and little specific data to support its thesis. Peltzman could not name any drug which had not been approved in the United States, and which his analysis showed should have been approved, when he was asked to do so during testimony before the Senate Subcommittee on Monopoly, March 14, 1973. Rather he replied, "I'm not prepared to get into names of drugs. I am more conservative than Professor Friedman, and so I recognize my limitations as a pharmacologist."[33] This, of course, did not enhance his credibility, even though his analysis was good.

Thus I could strengthen earlier arguments given at the end of the first NADC meeting which I attended on September 28, 1972:

> The [Dripps] Committee is really talking about economic priorities . . . because of . . . regulation . . . drug companies, in order to make money, are putting their research into products which they are more sure will be approved and that unfortunately . . . the [controlled] or

---

33. U.S. Senate, Select Committee on Small Business, Subcommittee on Monopoly, March 14, 1973, *Transcript,* pp. 10036, 10037.

double-blind or provable studies are far more difficult in the areas where we think the priorities of research belong.

And I ended with:

I think we ought to explore it [the effect of U.S. regulation of drugs] far beyond what we have done today.[34]

At that point Dr. Simmons requested that the discussion be "off-the-record."

Somewhat earlier during that same meeting, I had asked Dr. Simmons, "Do I read you that if you cannot construct a [controlled] double-blind study . . . [and] I conceive there may be some cases where you couldn't, then the drug cannot be approved?" Dr. Simmons replied: "There are some who would read the law that way. And that is where, you know, an agency has to be left some judgment to say 'all right, in this imperfect world that is the second best thing we can do in the public interest.' . . ."[35] (Transcript, p. 123)

By the winter of 1972, some of the major questions involved in the drug lag issue had been discussed by the NADC. For example: To what degree are significant new drugs not available in the United States but are available abroad? What are the criteria for a "significant" new drug? What is "substantial evidence"—only controlled, clinical studies done in the United States? and/or similar foreign studies? and/or foreign experience with the drugs marketed abroad?

In regard to the latter question the Supreme Court decision in *Weinberger* v. *Hynson, Westcott & Dunning* (1972) upheld "substantial evidence" as defined by section 505(d) of the act to include

> evidence consisting of adequate and well-controlled investigations, including clinical investigations, by experts qualified by scientific training and experience to evaluate the effectiveness of the drug involved. . . . Finally the regulation provides that "[u]ncontrolled studies or partially controlled studies are not acceptable as the *sole* [italics added] basis for the approval of claims of effectiveness. Such studies, carefully conducted and documented, may provide corroborative support. . . ."[36]

Thus evidence other than controlled clinical trials can be used as supportive evidence.

In early November 1972, I had written FDA for various materials to help resolve my thinking about whether and to what degree a drug lag may exist and what changes in FDA procedures could be made to speed up approvals

---

34. NADC *Transcript,* September 28, 1972, pp. 170, 171.
35. Ibid., p. 123.
36. U.S. Supreme Court, *Weinberger* v. *Hynson, Westcott and Dunning* (1972), 412 U.S. 609, pp. 609, 618.

while still meeting the safety and efficacy criteria. Dr. Simmons answered February 8, 1973, a few days after his lengthy testimony and that of Dr. Edwards before the Senate Subcommittee on Monopoly on February 5, 1973, in part as follows:

> . . . our data indicate that new drug applications approved in the past year have required an average of 30.5 months after the final receipt to receive approval. . . .
>
> The FDA regulations permit considerable support of a new drug application to come from foreign-generated clinical data. The only stipulation with respect to clinical trials is that at least some trials be performed in the United States, unless the disease being studied is rare or nonexistent in the United States. There is need, however, to develop guidelines for foreign drug studies which can be uniformly applied by both FDA and industry. These include such considerations as (1) qualifications of acceptable investigators; (2) monitoring studies by the firm; (3) peer review committees in institutions in which clinical trials are being performed; (4) the type of informed consent that may be acceptable; and (5) even such items as who legitimizes the translation of foreign case report forms and what reference drugs would be considered acceptable in controlled trials.
>
> Guidelines are currently in the process of development. This should increase our ability to utilize expertise wherever it exists. . . .
>
> There are no international agreements in this area at this time. . . .
>
> (Does FDA consider various cost-benefit ratios in its premarketing test requirements?)
>
> This is done only in the gross sense that we do not knowingly request industry to submit meaningless data or perform dubious studies. . . .[37]

Although FDA regulations may have permitted "considerable support" for an NDA from foreign data, the fact that an FDA regulation was proposed on September 6, 1973, and adopted May 9, 1975, to permit this, and that no guidelines for acceptance of data from foreign controlled studies existed until then, indicates that foreign data were little used.

On February 6, 1973, Dr. David P. Rutstein of the Harvard Medical School testified before the Senate Subcommittee on Monopoly that testing for the pharmacological characteristics of a new drug in a normal individual, after pretesting in animals for toxicity and indication of therapeutpc efficacy, is not always needed and raises ethical problems as compared to testing in patients who have the disease that the drug is designed to combat. He commented further that there is worldwide a waste of resources, unnecessary

---

37. Letter to Dr. Rita Campbell, February 8, 1973.

exposure of normal human subjects to the risks of drug testing, and delay in approving drugs here because of the lack of international collaborative agreements on both pre and postmarketing of drugs.[38]

Role of the Economist[39]

During committee meetings, I had expressed astonishment that computer searches of foreign literature on drugs were not routinely made, that foreign clinical data were not generally accepted, that well designed tests had to be repeated in the United States, and that U.S. firms could market a new drug abroad without informing the FDA of their intention to market abroad a drug for which they did or did not have an IND. The proposed regulation of September 6, 1973, stated that "an IND is not required when an investigational drug is manufactured and studied abroad [but] the FDA will accept one on a voluntary basis."[40] In order to circumvent having to apply for an IND to complete clinical studies within the United States, it appeared that some American companies had begun to shift some of their early research, as well as development of their new drugs, abroad. This meant that the United States was not benefiting as quickly as it might from all research by all the American pharmaceutical companies. Whether this delay was a necessary price for greater assurance of safety and efficacy might in 1972 still have been debatable. What surprised me was that FDA appeared to be unaware that there might be a loss in U.S. therapeutic medicine which the law and FDA's rigorous interpretation had induced.

Early in the morning of June 29, 1973, Dr. Richard Crout asked if he could look at my prepared notes for the brief presentation which FDA had asked me to give during that day's NADC meeting. Later that morning Dr. Marion Finkel announced, as if in answer to the first part of my intended presentation, that foreign literature computer searches would be routinely made; FDA would issue guidelines for acceptance of foreign clinical data; FDA would request U.S. firms to apply for an NDA simultaneously with an overseas application, whether or not they had an IND here; and FDA would cooperate fully with other countries in addition to World Health Organization (WHO) worldwide reporting of adverse drug data. For example, FDA would explore

---

38. David P. Rutstein, statement in U.S. Senate, Select Committee on Small Business, Subcommittee on Monopoly, February 6, 1973, mimeo, pp. 4, 6, 7.
39. Because this monograph is concerned with the drug lag and the role of the NADC, there is no discussion of drug prices, government reimbursement procedures, nor profits of pharmaceutical companies.
40. *Federal Register*, September 6, 1973, p. 24220.

premarket collaborative drug testing programs with other industrially advanced nations which have acceptable standards of drug testing.

My six pages of notes for the June 29 meeting detail why I believed that there was a drug lag. The primary table showed that from 1951 to 1962, an eleven-year period, the average annual number of new chemical entities introduced in the United States was 41.5, while from 1963-1970, the average annual number was only 16.1.[41] I commented further, and in part, that:

> The rate of slowdown of introduction or actual marketing of new drugs appears to be considerably greater than the rate of slowdown of discoveries of new drugs. There may be a lag in adjustment to the anticipated decrease in profits as costs increase from more test requirements of greater complexity. Several hypotheses may be explored to explain this . . . .

> New drugs, it may be argued, are not *per se* always a good thing. But new drugs which have been successfully marketed over a period of years in an industrially advanced country are meeting a medical need. The patient, in conjunction with his physician, prefers them to substitutes. Other factors as well as the 1962 amendment are involved in the slowing of the rate of introduction of new drugs in the United States. . . [My copy of the official transcript of the June 29, 1973 meeting of NADC does not have a page 3. The preceding paragraph was on that missing page, according to my typed notes.]

> It is easier to assess *post facto,* the degree of harm caused by a non-safe drug than to estimate before the fact the potential loss of benefit from an efficacious, relatively safe drug being withheld from the market. This makes policy decisions in this area difficult. Few people have tried to estimate such potential losses of benefit. . . .

> It seems to me that one of the biggest problems in policymaking is that there are different classifications of risks and benefits in relationship to drugs. This is because there are four variables: size of potential risk, number of potential persons who may bear the risk, size of potential benefit, and number of people who might benefit. . . .

> The criteria for establishing efficacy and safety are different where there is potentially high risk to many persons and potentially small benefit to a few persons as compared to a low risk, great benefit to many persons drug. In fact, it is probable that the manufacturer has already screened out of the market drugs that fall within the high risk, small benefit to a few persons, type of classification. It would seem to me that in some way the criteria which are set for acceptability of a new drug should have

---

41. E. Reis-Arndt and D. Elvers, "Results of Pharma Research: New Pharmaceutical Agents 1961-1970," in *Drugs Made in Germany,* vol. 5, no. 3 (Ingelheim, West Germany: C.H. Boehringer Sohn, 1972), p. 135.

> some relationship to the particular risk/benefit ratio involved. The FDA has recognized this when it approved L-Dopa prior to full completion of Phase III studies, where there is a high risk to few persons and potentially a very great benefit to the same few people. In other words, when the alternatives or options to the patient or consumer are such that he is willing to take a large risk for a large benefit, such an option should be open to him. This is an area of value judgments and not necessarily only the domain of a government body composed of the pharmacologist, the physician, and the clinical research scientist . . .

I ended with three questions:

> How can the United States utilize the statistical experience of large numbers of persons using a new drug in a foreign country? Where controlled tests meeting ethical standards are difficult to devise, foreign experience is of greater importance. . . .

> In what ways can criteria for marketing be tailored to the different risk/benefit classes as suggested above? . . .

> Can postmarket review of drugs be improved so as to know more precisely the probability of what percent of those receiving a drug will find the drug to be efficacious, toxic, or neutral? As I understand it, the adverse reporting program is entirely voluntary on the part of physicians. . . . Therefore, there is no reporting of when it's beneficial . . . it's not feasible to assume that the reporting is complete . . . you start looking for data which do not exist. . . . You don't know what percentage of the dosages are toxic and which are efficacious.

My presentation and ensuing discussion revealed that I had much to learn, but at the same time it did make clear that economists also had something to offer. The assumption that the United States has all the expert scientists who conduct the technically excellent and ethically acceptable clinical drug studies appeared to me, working at an internationally staffed research institution, a bit provincial. Additionally, the U.S. policy of approving drugs much later than other countries permits other nations to charge the United States with using their populations to serve as guinea pigs—a practice somewhat open to ethical criticism. For example, Dr. Richard Crout was reported to have told the Drug Experience Advisory Committee meeting, September 13:

> Many, if not most, new molecules appearing in the U.S. today, are already being marketed in Europe. I don't know how long this trend will continue but it may well be. . .at least another decade. . . .We ought to be able to have an early warning system for severe drug reactions, particularly those that occur early in the marketing experience. . . .It may be that the best way to do this is to rely on European data.[42]

---

42. *FDC Reports,* "The Pink Sheet," T&G-2, September 16, 1974.

The lack of agreement of so-called hard data of the effects of a given drug meant to several other committee members and to me that biostatisticians were underutilized, and even when used, the judgments of the policymakers as to which are the more reliable data still often reflect value judgments rather than compelling conclusions that the data mandate.

The degree of nonagreement of results among studies done by reputable scientists, the intensity of controversy over the meaning of conflicting data, and the "correct" interpretation of a single set of data surprised me. For years, experts in the so-called "hard sciences" have criticized social scientists for their soft data and economists especially for their publicized disagreements over interpretation of existing data and extrapolation of future trends. That biology, pharmacology, epidemiology, and medicine generally also did not have simple, agreed-upon data leading to defensible conclusions, I had long suspected, but the intensity of some of the disagreement was a surprise.

The lack of conclusive, reliable data, in-house as well as among its advisory committees, may be the major reason why FDA has interpreted "substantial evidence" of efficacy to mean almost always "two double-blind, placebo-controlled clinical studies" which are in substantial agreement as to outcomes, before granting approval of a new drug application. FDA has at times waived these requirements and tailored them to the particular risk/benefit relationship involved: for example, in the case of cancer drugs where the outcome without treatment is a high probability of death, the risk acceptable to the patient is assumed to be very high.

Despite this, Adriamycin, "which has a very broad spectrum of activity in cancer," was originally approved abroad in 1971 and in this country only in August 1974—the thirty-second country to do so.[43] Dr. Zubrod suggested, during testimony before a Senate subcommittee, that when a drug for cancer is on sale in England and has gone through screening by the British Dunlop Committee, ". . .a panel on cancer at the FDA might look at the data from Italy and England and see whether or not a limited type of NDA might be in order at this point." Even though the Cancer Institute does use it throughout their research network, "the drug reaches only a small fraction of those patients who could benefit from it."[44]

Dr. Zubrod also stated that even when the U.S. Government has done all the research on a cancer drug and offers it to a company under an exclusive license, there would be "3 or 4 years, before it moved from the time experts said we should make this generally available and the time at which this actually will be accomplished, with the filing of an NDA." Dr. Zubrod

---

43. Zubrod, op. cit., p. 9678.
44. Ibid., pp. 9678, 9679.

explained that "the preparation of an NDA and marketing is expensive" and further that there are delays in filing for NDAs because there is a type of ". . .foreign sponsor who simply does not wish to apply for an NDA in this country. . .[and] with drugs that are found to have a second usage there [are] the difficulties in getting the labeling changed for the second usage and the companies may not wish to file."[45]

A New FDA Commissioner

Although subsequent meetings of NADC touched on issues peripheral to drug lag, the general issue was never brought up again at an NADC meeting. Alexander Schmidt, M.D., Dean of the School of Medicine, University of Illinois, was appointed FDA commissioner prior to the June 1973 meeting. The October 11-12, 1973 meeting was, however, the first meeting which Dr. Schmidt chaired. At that meeting he and Dr. Edwards, then HEW's Assistant Secretary for Health, set FDA's functions within HEW's, and HEW's functions were defined as set by the requirements of the Office of Management and Budget (OMB). The main emphasis appeared to be that FDA must respond to OMB's guidelines for justification of FDA programs within the overall U.S. budget allocations. Specific goals and a cost-benefit approach to select the best means to reach a goal were highlighted. Although this was a general approach, it was clear that a cost-benefit analysis to answer whether a therapeutic drug lag existed could be fitted into this framework.

At the end of a speech significantly entitled, "Dimensions of Change in FDA," the new FDA Commissioner Schmidt referred to a "drug development gap" and stated, September 13, 1973, that "the evidence I have discovered to date simply doesn't support the view that Americans are being denied valuable new drugs because of FDA bumbling, procrastination or for any other reason. . . .we are getting the expert opinion of others and should be able to give the public a more definitive answer in the future. *I will change my mind as the facts might require. . . .* [italics added]"[46]

Although in many respects other statements within this speech may be of greater general importance, the new commissioner's continuing commitment to take a new look at the questions, whether they involved informed consent by the patient, package insert labels for prescription medicines for patients with chronic disease, or advertising and pricing of drugs, was a new approach

---

45. Ibid., pp. 9676, 9677.
46. Alexander Schmidt, "Dimensions of Change in the FDA," speech before the Pharmaceutical Advertising Seminar, Chicago, September 13, 1973, mimeo, p. 4.

for FDA and one which meant change. Dr. Schmidt announced that he would consider all sides of a "dialogue" and would seek "the specifics of change and the needed commitments to change."[47]

With Dr. Schmidt's appointment, FDA's policy in respect to the drug lag charge began to change, and approvals of drugs already in the pipeline also began to emerge. Some of these changes had already been foreshadowed by Simmons and Finkel under Edwards. When Edwards became Assistant Secretary for Health, Henry Simmons moved with him and Richard Crout became Director of the Bureau of Drugs.

On September 6, 1973, the *Federal Register* carried the FDA proposal to accept clinical data on new drugs generated outside the United States which began with the following "Peter's Preamble"[48]: "The Commissioner of Food and Drugs is concerned over the loss in the new drug approval process in the United States of clinical data from studies performed by experts abroad. . ." and therefore permits "inclusion of studies performed outside of this country . . . [in order] to further the availability to the American public in a timely fashion of important new drugs being studied abroad." The proposal would request international manufacturers to submit data for drug approval to the FDA simultaneously with submission of data for approval by a foreign country. The proposal became regulation which has the impact of law on May 9, 1975.[49]

Dr. Schmidt recognized that all the benefits from a drug, for example an increase in food supply which results from adding the chemical DES to cattle feed, must be weighed against the degree and probability of adverse effects or risks and other costs of the same drug. The committee which initially was charged "to advise and consult. . .to review and evaluate Agency programs" was encouraged to evolve primarily as a sounding board on such important public questions as the nature of the ethics involved in drug experimentation on humans in the testing of new drugs: use of normal children and prisoners in new drug trials, nature of informed consent, confidentiality, and reasonable length of follow-up of subjects. Meeting time was largely utilized by the FDA staff for extensive briefings, leaving little time for input by members. FDA's usual practice during 1972 and 1973 was not to mail out material relevant to the subject prior to the meetings. A new executive secretary for NADC, the committee's main liaison with FDA, and changes in the top level of FDA, in

---

47. Ibid., p. 15.
48. "Peter's Preambles" refer to carefully worded "preambles" by Peter Hutt, FDA's general counsel, which justified with bibliographical citations most of Commissioner Schmidt's "Regulations."
49. *Federal Register,* April 9, 1975, pp. 16053-57.

addition to objections from the committee,[50] brought about a gradual change in this practice.

It was the understanding of at least one member of NADC ". . .that the Committee was appointed not only to have some input, but also to bear some responsibility and take some of the criticism off the FDA."[51] This was not substantially different from FDA's original concept of NADC's main function, as indicated after the off-the-record discussion of September 28, 1972, by Dr. Simmons as follows:

> What Dr. Edwards asked us to do tomorrow was to try to get this committee in the very short time available conversant with the way things are done on the drug side of the agency. After all, you're going to be the National Advisory Drug Council [sic] you have to know, trust, and believe in the system before you can be advocates.[52]

Whether NADC's initial refusal to issue a definitive statement concerning drug lag and their insistence on first hearing from Dr. Dripps and others influenced this remark, I do not know, but the NADC was never again asked to issue a statement on this or indeed on any other matter, although at times votes were sought, and NADC's discussions acted as a buffer.

During the spring and summer of 1973, considerable correspondence by the NADC members was circulated among them on the "Use of Advisory Committees in Drug Evaluation." This was in response to FDA's request, because they were planning to expand, when OMB preferred that they contract, the number of "expert" advisory committees primarily because in-house expertise appeared to be lacking in many areas, an easily understandable fact given the relatively low salaries and recent testimony as to conditions of work.[53] Additionally, an investigation by a congressional oversight committee might have been anticipated in view of the Federal Advisory Committee Act signed into law October 6, 1972.

Part of the NADC internal correspondence discusses how such committees

---

50. For example, Merrill Hines, M.D. (Medical Director, Ochsner Clinic), wrote to the executive secretary, Dr. Albert Esch, October 5, 1972: "I feel very strongly that better communication between the FDA and the National Advisory Drug Committee would be useful." Further, V.S. Burnham commented in an August 16, 1973 memorandum to all NADC members and FDA staff: "Often we have the impression we are working in a vacuum without specific information in regard to certain subjects discussed or assigned to us to report upon. Both Dr. Campbell and Mr. Smith bring this point out."

51. Hines letter, ibid.

52. NADC *Transcript,* September 28, 1972, p. 176.

53. *Report on Use of Advisory Committees in Drug Regulation,* M.J. Finkel, Chairman, March 5, 1973: "We now have twelve (plus the Biometry and Epidemiology Committee) and anticipate that sixteen or perhaps eighteen will be the final total." Mimeo.

can better deal with benefit/risk ratios. FDA policy was that NDAs with "narrow benefit/risk ratios" should be among those brought before advisory committees. With this NADC agreed.

Dr. Schmidt first chaired an NADC meeting in October 1973, only a few weeks after his receipt of the Dripps Committee letter of September 24, 1973, which contained the following significant paragraphs:

> We were encouraged to read on the occasion of your taking office that while you believe in the need for regulation for public safety, you will be looking at the balance between regulation and the need to avoid inhibiting R&D. This question of maximizing benefit to patients has been the central concern of our group.
>
> We have also been encouraged to see that in the last two months FDA has cleared several important compounds which have long been available overseas. We would like to point out, however, that the timing of these FDA actions supports our belief that the U.S. has fallen behind the rest of the world. For these four compounds, the average time between NDA submission and approval in the U.S. was almost five years. Also, on the average, they were introduced into the U.S. almost eight years after being introduced in Britain. . . .
>
> We suspect that the delays seen with these compounds are not isolated cases but confirm the existence of a real drug lag. It is also significant to note that these four compounds originated with foreign owned firms and were initially marketed in foreign countries.

To Commissioner Schmidt the main function of the NADC appeared to be a sounding board in order to judge how the public in general might react to various FDA proposals. This function might have been better performed by a body more representative of the general public. Among the subjects discussed at the October 1973 meeting and those later in 1974 were drug labeling; whether informative leaflets should be inserted in some prescription drug packages for patient use; role of the pharmacist; advertising of prices of prescription drugs; bioavailability of generic and brand name drugs—but not the drug lag. There were only two meetings actually held in 1974, in January and April. Consensus rather than actual vote was usually, but not always, sought by the commissioner chairman.

FDA Considers Cost-Benefit Analysis

Meanwhile, I had been asked by Dr. Lloyd Tepper, Associate Commissioner for Science, FDA, to write a brief paper explaining as simply as possible—no equations—cost-benefit analysis and its uses and limitations in policy decisions on food safety. The paper was officially for

> ...a compendium of materials relevant to a possible modification of the Delaney Clause... [because] we find that economic considerations are important in that substances barred under anti-cancer laws (such as certain growth promotants or preservatives) might expand the food supply to our great economic advantage. Accordingly we should like to have a section on economics in the compendium defining how economic principles are utilized in risk-benefit considerations....[54]

Unofficially, the study was also used to educate FDA's staff as to how economists think. The original study was published under the title *Food Safety Regulation: A Study of the Use and Limitations of Cost-Benefit Analysis* by the Hoover Institution and American Enterprise Institute (AEI) in August 1974. An abbreviated version of my original paper was printed earlier as part of the FDA Compendium on the Delaney Clause in the U.S. House of Representatives, Subcommittee on Appropriations, *Hearings,* Part 8, *FDA: Study of the Delaney Clause and other Anti-Cancer Clauses,* under the title "Appraisal of Benefit: The Economists' Point of View."[55] Dr. Schmidt explained that FDA

> made a serious effort to enlist the collaboration of a spectrum of people who are authorities in their respective fields and familiar with the problems of additives and carcinogenesis.
>
> This general approach was reviewed with your staff and deemed suitable to accomplish the objectives outlined by the committee.
>
> Each identified participant was invited to contribute material in his or her assigned area. We were pleased to receive excellent cooperation, although, as you can imagine, since busy people who are authorities in highly technical areas have great demands upon their time, there was a certain amount of slippage, none of great consequence. Each contribution, with two exceptions, was edited so as to achieve some similarity of technical level and format. Contributors were told, however, that they are free to publish their material as papers in scientific journals or other media, so that you may eventually see or become aware of more extended discussion of the topics addressed in the compilation.[56]

All names of the authors were separated from their writings in that government publication and abbreviated biographies of each contributor were alphabetically listed.

---

54. Letter to Dr. Rita Campbell, September 24, 1973.

55. U.S. House of Representatives, Committee on Appropriations, Subcommittee on Agriculture-Environmental and Consumer Protection, *Hearings,* Part 8, May 6, 1974, pp. 437-89.

56. Ibid., pp. 25, 26.

Pressures on FDA

Concurrent with the drug lag charge, internal and external pressures were exerted against FDA to withdraw existing approvals and not approve other new drugs. This culminated on August 15, 1974 when eleven present and past FDA employees and three consultants stated before a joint hearing of the Senate Subcommittee on Health and the Senate Administrative Practice Subcommittee that they were harassed and some reassigned when they advised against approving drugs.

Discontent among the professional staff had been building since the second physical move of FDA within six years, this time from Crystal City, Virginia to the Parklawn Building in Rockville, Maryland in 1970. Dr. Edwards became commissioner in 1969, the fourth commissioner in a six-year period, and he tried to develop managerial systems out of a chaotic situation. In the words of Dr. Crout, who testified April 19, 1976 before the Chalmers Review Panel on New Drug Regulations about the drug review process:

> First, to get hold of the document control system, a task force, of which I was head, was appointed early in 1972. It consisted of scientific people and our consumer safety officers and others as parts of a document control team. It took two years, but as a result we instituted a document control system and a new management control system, whereby it's all on computers, which indicate who gets what document and what the time limits are on it, and so on. It might be a little astounding to know that wasn't known before, but it wasn't. Prior to 1974 not one scientific officer in our place knew his work assignments, nor did any manager know work assignments of people under him. Now the next part of that concept was that once you get documents under control, you can rationally build, even rationally allocate them where they should be allocated. We were already arranged in divisions, six divisions. Those divisions were unbalanced in their size, so another thrust was made to equalize the divisions, and to put three groups in each division. This is entirely medical officers, who were assigned to clusters.[57]

The most extraordinary part of Crout's testimony, however, was his description of FDA's breakdown in line authority stemming from the "managerial style" of past Commissioner Dr. Goddard:

> During his tenure line management tended to break down. Channels of reporting tended to be more personal, that is reporting to Dr. Goddard personally. That, combined with the moves, the reorganization, left line management disastrously weak by the late 1960s. Nobody wanted to be

---

57. Unofficial, non-edited thermographic copy of Richard Crout's testimony, pp. 5, 6.

manager. I'll tell you that in my first year at the FDA, and even lasting longer than that into [19]72-73, going to certain kinds of meetings was an extraordinarily peculiar kind of exercise. People—and I'm talking about division directors and their staffs, engaged in a kind of behavior that invited insubordination. There were people tittering in corners, throwing spitballs. I'm describing physicians. There were people who slouched down in a chair and did not respond to questions, moaned and groaned with sweeping gestures. A kind of behavior I have not seen in any other institution as a grown man. Now that's the kind of morale and the kind of organization problems with which the Parklawn Building began.[58]

Dr. Edwards restored normal line management controls which involved a major reorganization. The resulting transfers of physicians peaked in 1974 with transfers from FDA's cardiovascular division to other divisions in order to gain balance of personnel and tasks and to implement the "concept that drugs and drug experts should be brought together."[59] Some of the persons who were transferred complained to Ralph Nader's Health Research Group and then to Senator Kennedy, who chaired the joint hearing mid-August of 1974. Meanwhile, from time to time the Health Research Group of Ralph Nader's Consumer Advocacy Group protested in testimony on the Hill and before NADC meetings that there was a lack of protection of consumers, that consumers were allowed to waste money on ineffective drugs, and also that informed consent procedures for institutionalized persons on whom experimental drugs were being tested were inadequate.

Commissioner Schmidt's 906-page mimeographed report on the eleven FDA employees' charges was released October 24, 1975, and he stated, "my investigation has not only revealed no evidence to support such general charges, it has produced evidence to refute those charges—evidence long available."[60] Dr. Crout testified on September 27, 1974, that "there were no approvals in the cardiovascular area in the years between 1967 and 1972," thus upholding Dr. Wardell's previous comment in relation to the charge that employees were forced towards a bias in favor of drug approvals: "I cannot see how some of these people can have approved drugs because there were not any approved."[61]

A review panel headed by Thomas C. Chalmers, M.D., was appointed by

---

58. Ibid., p. 3.
59. Ibid., p. 6.
60. Alexander Schmidt, *The Commissioner's Report of Investigation of Charges,* October 1975, mimeo, p. 894.
61. U.S. Senate, Committee on Labor and Public Welfare, Subcommittee on Health, *Transcript,* pp. 69, 70.

HEW Secretary Weinberger to explore further these complaints of FDA personnel and to assess the commissioner's report. The original charge was expanded from investigating maladministration by FDA to a study of existing policies and procedures for the regulation of new drugs by FDA. The review panel reported May 1976 only on *Assessment of the Commissioner's Report of October 1975* and did not review the far more important issue from the point of view of the public: the effect of government regulation on introduction of new drugs in the United States and how this process might, with continued assurance of safety and efficacy to the consumer, be speeded up. The seven-person panel had a staff of ten persons, including seven lawyers and one physician, but apparently only one economist on temporary loan.

The prestigious *New England Journal of Medicine* decried both the commissioner's 906-page report and the Chalmers Committee's 525-page critique, noting that the chairman, Dr. Chalmers, dissented from his own committee's report and resigned from the panel in June 1976. Subsequently Lionel Bernstein, M.D., Executive Secretary, was reassigned to other duties by HEW Secretary David Mathews. That the panel's staff numbered ten and the committee only seven, and members of the latter of course were busy at their regular jobs and therefore were available on only a very limited part-time basis, gives credence to Chalmer's dissenting statement that "it became apparent to the chairman that the technique adopted by the staff of listing every conceivable criticism in the draft analyses could lead to the prejudicial final document." More important, however, it so absorbed the panel's resources that it make it impossible "to conduct a broad review of current policies and procedures of new drug regulation."[62] Thus an in-depth discussion of whether drugs were being released too rapidly or too slowly was avoided and David Greenberg's scathing review in the *New England Journal of Medicine* seems warranted: "The panelists for all their prestige and professional accomplishments have turned out to be a bickering lot of hair splitting metaphysicians, and if HEW Secretary David Mathews chooses to sweep them all out, it will be no loss to the Republic on drug safety and efficacy."[63] Secretary Mathews' letter of June 4, 1976, actually appears to accomplish this end because it terminates the panel September 30, 1976:

> I believe it appropriate for the Panel not to participate in further investigation of these allegations, but now to turn its efforts to the general issues facing the Food and Drug Administration. The Panel can

---

62. U.S. HEW, Review Panel on New Drug Regulations, *Assessment of the Commissioner's Report of October 1975,* May 1976, mimeo, p. 52.
63. *New England Journal of Medicine,* vol. 294, no. 26, p. 1465.

draw upon the reservoir of information gained from the investigation of specific allegations as well as from its other efforts and devote the time remaining until the Panel's September 30 termination date to provide specific advice on ways to improve new drug regulation policies and procedures, and to identify problem areas that require future study. . . . Commissioner Schmidt, Assistant Secretary Cooper and I believe it is of the utmost importance to identify ways in which the Food and Drug Administration can improve its regulation of new drugs. The magnitude and complexity of its regulatory activities are so great that a series of improvements may be expected to evolve over a period of years.[64]

Secretary Mathews, however, after further Kennedy hearings in mid-July, was persuaded to extend the life of the panel to March 31, 1977.

If the aim is, as that letter states, to improve FDA's regulation of new drugs, I believe that a new panel with a more balanced representation—three of the seven-member Chalmers Panel are lawyers and four are physicians or scientists—is needed.

Probably the greatest pressure on FDA comes from congressional hearings and persons on the Hill. In the calendar year 1973, top FDA officials participated in twenty-three congressional hearings, sixteen of which dealt with drugs, including similar problems such as pesticides and ozone layers, but not including foods, cosmetics, budget, and use of advisory committees. In 1974, the respective figures were thirty-two hearings, seventeen specifically on drugs, and as of November 3, 1975, actual and probable hearings in open and executive session appeared to be increasing in number.[65]

In January 1976, the House Government Operations Committee charged in an oversight report abuses in FDA's use of advisory committees and that FDA ". . .uses such committees as 'window dressing' to gain physician support for its decisions and to dilute its responsibility for effective regulation of the drug industry."[66] Also during January 1976 the General Accounting Office criticized FDA for inadequate oversight of drug testing on humans.[67]

As I have written elsewhere, adverse effects of drugs are publicized while potential benefits of an unapproved drug are not generally known.[68] This prejudices decision making to support the *status quo*—not to "rock the boat." The FDA commissioner almost always treads a delicate line between Scylla

---

64. David Mathew's letter to Thomas C. Chalmers, June 4, 1976.
65. U.S. HEW, Listing of all hearings the Food and Drug Administration has participated in from 1973 to date, March 26, 1975, and subsequent reports, mimeo.
66. *Congressional Quarterly,* January 31, 1976, p. 223. House Report 94-787, January 26, 1976.
67. *Congressional Quarterly,* January 31, 1976, p. 224.
68. Campbell, op. cit., pp. 22 ff.

and Charybdis situations. The law for example does not define what is "an imminent hazard to the public health" but the FDA commissioner may remove drugs summarily whenever the commissioner believes that this phrase applies. "Imminent hazard to the public health" needs to be defined by statute, as, for example, a "high probability of serious risk" and the latter, if it is an acceptable definition, be defined further to indicate what is *high* probability and *serious* risk. That political and publicity pressures will overcome logical analysis, however, I do not believe has to be the general case if the commissioner, as Dr. Schmidt has demonstrated, is astute and courageous enough to stand up for what he believes.[69] Such a commissioner can use advisory committees to support his analytically sound positions and might overcome, with aid from others, the built-in conservative bias of a *status quo* situation which the Sunshine Acts and publicity build into decisions involving future risk taking.

Other organized pressure groups have been the American Medical Association, various associations of pharmacists, the National Association of Retail Druggists, the Pharmaceutical Manufacturers' Association, and the Health Research Group of Ralph Nader. The last of these does not really represent the consumer, but rather the interests of a professional consumer advocate. Consumer advocacy groups may originate from a given issue about which they feel strongly and which they have intensively researched, an approach which is almost a necessity if they are to continue to receive financial support to ensure their existence. As consumer advocacy groups spread their attentions over a greater number of issues, the quality of their research becomes diluted. Since the financial support of consumer advocacy groups comes from persons who believe in the issues which they espouse, such groups tend to support the more easily explained and publicized position on issues rather than the more complicated, often less emotional position. Adverse effects from marketed drugs rather than loss of benefits from unapproved drugs, about which the public may have little idea, fit ideally into this pattern, and the literature indicates that the true public interest appears to be in the less flamboyant area. The longer a consumer advocacy group exists the more likely it is, if financially self-supporting, to be run like a business.

Pressure by organized groups is more effective than by unorganized groups. The NADC spent many hours discussing how FDA might get more effective

---

69. In a recent article (which I understand is to be published) read after the draft of this monograph was written, David Seidman of the Social Science Research Council stated in a case study of drug lag: "But the FDA does not attempt to measure the costs and benefits," and "Congress appears to be almost totally impervious to systematic policy analysis." Seidman, "Protection and Overprotection, the Politics and Economics of Pharmaceutical Regulation," paper given at Midwest Political Science Association, April 29-May 1, 1976, mimeo, pp. 22, 28.

consumer input. Although NADC noted that any person with expertise outside (as well as inside) of the direct area being regulated was also a consumer as well as an expert in his profession, this would probably not result in all socio-economic classes being represented. The NADC did recommend that all FDA scientific committees have at least one statistician. Some members felt that general advisory committees, such as the NADC, should also have a lawyer as well as an economist on these and possibly other FDA committees. Some members thought that at least one "not-at-interest" consumer should be a voting, paid member on many of FDA's committees.[70]

As Commissioner Schmidt has remarked:

> Facing the reality that life involves risk and that no amount of government regulation can remove all risk, then how much risk does the public find acceptable—especially in the use of therapeutic chemicals which all have potential for harm as well as benefit?[71]

To answer such questions as these, opinions of persons not at interest should be considered.

FDA's Position on Drug Lag Changes

On September 27, 1974, the head of the Bureau of Drugs, Dr. Crout, stated:

> The data cited by Dr. Wardell are correct. There were no approvals in hypertensive drugs in the first decade after the amendments. There were no approvals in the cardiovascular area in the years between 1967 and 1972, and that is the fact of life and is one of the causes of much of the concern by physicians and so on about the drug lag business. That is one of the causes of the formation of committees and everything else. It is fairly evident from reading the literature that that segment was disparate from the drug approval process compared with the rate of approvals in other areas. The data are correct. . . .The. . .gap. . .was limited to the cardiovascular and pulmonary [area].[72]

---

70. FDA advisory review panels on over-the-counter or nonprescription drugs do have usually one non-voting and non-paid consumer member who may be selected from organized consumer groups such as the Consumer Federation of America. When the consumer is the only non-voting and non-paid member, his opinion is downgraded by some of the other members. Selection of non-paid consumers is limited in practice from persons who live in the Washington, D.C. area and from those who can afford to give daytime hours for public service. This means that retired persons and homemakers without children below school age are most likely to be selected as members.

71. Schmidt, "Dimensions of Change in the FDA," p. 9.

72. U.S. Senate, Joint Hearings: Committee on Labor and Public Welfare—Subcommittee on Health, and Committee on Judiciary—Subcommittee on Administrative Practice and Procedure, *Transcript,* September 27, 1974, mimeo, pp. 69, 70.

Commissioner Schmidt's testimony dated August 16, 1974 stated:

> In sum, it is clear that the rate of drug introduction into the United States has slowed since the 1950's. This slowdown is worldwide, but is somewhat greater in this country than in other advanced countries. There appear to be some drugs unavailable in this country that represent modest but real therapeutic gains. We are concerned about this and want to be very sure that useful drugs are not held back unnecessarily. It also appears that drug research has moved abroad to some extent. We are also concerned about this, because of its negative impact on the development of good clinical investigation in therapeutics and because it will further delay the availability of useful drugs.[73]

And on October 29, 1974, Commissioner Schmidt, in what might be considered a plea for a positive rather than a negative legislative mandate to the FDA, spoke at the National Press Club as follows:

> What I see as a seriously unbalanced and deleterious pressure can be remedied only by Congressional and public recognition that the *failure* to approve an important new drug can be as detrimental to the public health as the approval of a potentially bad drug. It's often forgotten—and sometimes conveniently so—that our responsibility to get good new drugs into medical practice is at least as important as our responsibility to keep worthless or dangerous drugs off the market.[74]

Meanwhile, an improvement in FDA's approvals of NDAs had occurred between 1971 and 1976. In September 1974, Dr. William Wardell, their most effective critic because his criticism was based on primary scientific data and was reported in terms which FDA staff could more easily understand than criticism by economists, had stated before the Senate Subcommittee on Health:

> Over the past 2½ years, a marked improvement has occurred in the rate of FDA approvals of medically useful new drugs, with resulting benefits for the American patient. . . .Large anachronisms still remain—e.g., in the cardiovascular area. . . .Nevertheless, in general the FDA has come to be more in touch with up-to-date standards of medical practice, and has done much to regain the confidence of the scientific and medical communities. . . .[75]

---

73. Ibid., p. 28. Although dated August 16, 1974, was referred to September 25, 1974, several times but not actually orally presented during the hearings.
74. Alexander Schmidt, "The FDA Today: Critics, Congress, and Consumerism," speech before the National Press Club, mimeo, p. 12.
75. U.S. Senate, Joint Hearings, op. cit., September 27, 1974, p. 507.

Some clarification of the distinction between the scientific and the legal approaches and the difficulty in resolving them was achieved during the same hearing when Wardell commented regarding the disagreements on drug approvals as follows:

> Disagreements are in the nature of value judgments. This is an area which, in legal terms, is rather hard to define right or wrong. These are scientific areas still under discussion. I can give you my interpretation of the drugs. I certainly think that several things were not available, then subsequently. . .approved. For instance, Adriamycin, Cromolyn—these are obvious answers.[76]

On November 2, 1975, Senator Kennedy, who had queried Dr. Wardell during the Senate Subcommittee hearings of September 1974, stated that "There are fundamental defects in our nation's current regulatory procedures for prescription drugs. . .lack of any follow-up, once the drugs have reached the market." Although Senator Kennedy and Commissioner Schmidt may disagree on some aspects of causes and remedies, they apparently do agree that, in Senator Kennedy's words, "Badly needed drugs are delayed from joining the fight against disease," that the lack of post-market data does not protect the consumer because "the harmful true effects are not fully known," and that "the lack of follow-up also makes it difficult to discover new uses for existing drugs."[77]

On November 5, 1975, at the same Tulane medical symposium, Commissioner Schmidt suggested at least four major changes in FDA procedures, changes which had been discussed during meetings of the National Advisory Drug Committee: (1) early participation by FDA in the design of clinical studies; (2) "There should be a continued and sequential review of data submitted as part of an IND or NDA, so that at any given time, all interested parties know how the tally sheet reads;" (3) ". . .a more flexible approval process, coupled with a post marketing data collection system;" and (4) ". . .the ability to approve drugs for restricted uses; e.g., only in a hospital, only by certain specialists, or only by physicians who had taken a specific period of training or who would agree to report results in a particular manner." Dr. Schmidt summarized the anticipated effect as follows: ". . .these changes might permit earlier appearance in the United States of many drugs, in return for a longer investigational phase controlled by FDA.

---

76. Ibid., p. 47.
77. Edward Kennedy, "[Keynote] Address," press release of speech before the Tulane Medical Symposium on Principles and Techniques of Human Research and Therapeutics, New Orleans, November 2, 1975, mimeo, pp. 3, 4a.

This seems to me a reasonable trade-off. . . .[78]

Dr. Leo E. Hollister has succinctly described the FDA procedures which make needlessly long and costly the process followed to obtain permission to market a drug:

> A long hiatus occurs between the initial filing of the Notice of Investigational New Drug (IND) and the submission of the NDA. Customarily, it requires several resubmissions of the NDA before approval is granted, largely because of some afterthoughts on the part of FDA reviewers. As it may take up to 180 days to get each afterthought, and it may take months or years of work to answer each of these, the reason for the long process becomes obvious. It has been repeatedly suggested that the preparation of the NDA be planned at each successive phase of drug investigation prior to marketing by a joint group which would include the FDA reviewers, the pharmaceutical company sponsors, the clinical investigators testing the drug, and independent experts. . . .Once an acceptable set of plans had been agreed upon, they might be regarded in spirit, if not in law, as constituting a contract. Obviously, one would wish to have the right to make exceptions if some unusual finding arose in relation to the drug. Such a system would assure a continuing review of the developing NDA with the flexibility needed to prove the drug by the latest techniques of the clinic or the laboratory.[79]

The extraordinary number of pages of raw data required for an NDA, and the continuing increase in that bulk of paper in FDA's archives as scientific techniques become more complex and closer tolerances are reached, point to a need for reform of this regulatory process. A major current proposal, supported in various forms by Commissioner Schmidt, Senator Kennedy, and Professor Wardell, is to release new drugs earlier to specialists (or as some suggest, to all physicians who promise to meet special reporting requirements) and then greatly intensify post-market review in phase IV studies. This procedure has been used by FDA in the case of L-Dopa, Cromolyn Sodium, and Triazure.[80]

Another proposal is that certified summaries of the data from the clinical studies could be accepted instead of the raw data. This would greatly speed up the review process.

---

78. Alexander Schmidt, "The FDA in 1985," speech before the Tulane Medical Symposium, New Orleans, November 5, 1975, mimeo, p. 3.

79. Leo Hollister, "The FDA Ten Years After the Kefauver-Harris Amendment," *Perspectives in Biology and Medicine,* winter 1974, p. 244.

80. Although all approved new drugs are subject to post-marketing surveillance (21 CFR 310.300), FDA may also give an earlier approval under circumstances outlined in their new drug regulations (21 CFR 310.303) if the company agrees to conduct special studies and provide additional data, as from long-term studies.

What Was the Role of Cost-Benefit Analysis in the Drug Lag Issue?

In view of the obvious lack of data, cost-benefit analysis is difficult to use in assessing net societal benefits from a given drug. The better the drug in a biological sense, the easier to estimate its probable economic worth. Being currently involved in a prospective study on cost-benefit assessment of economic benefits from a new drug, I am acutely aware of the complications involved in these measurements.

The lack of definition of "public interest" in even the limited health sector of "drugs" makes comparative use of net benefits in policy decisions difficult. Probably the best definition I have seen is Wardell's: "Patients—and the rest of society as potential patients—have two main needs with respect to drugs: the development of improved (i.e., more effective or less toxic) drugs; and the better utilization of all drugs."[81]

To accomplish this goal, emphasis on protection of the consumer from harm by new drugs must be weighed against the probable loss of creative innovations that would result in new, therapeutically more effective drugs for the many diseases for which there are no effective drugs. Whether the shift of U.S. pharmaceutical research abroad even in the early stages by U.S. companies, to avoid having to go through the lengthy process of getting an IND, will be reversed if this approach to regulation is adopted, is not known. Commissioner Schmidt's recent statements give hope that it will be, but because it will be expensive for companies which have established research operations overseas to reverse their current policy, no such forecast can be made. Secondary economic effects, for example greater unemployment in the United States than otherwise, also cannot be overlooked.

The Food and Drug Administration had no economist during the period when policy on drug lag was being discussed by NADC, and as was the case with other regulatory agencies, FDA was not required to submit an inflation impact statement until April 1975, under Executive Order 11821, November 27, 1974.

As late as November 20, 1975, Gerald Barkdoll, FDA's Assistant Commissioner for Planning and Evaluation, spoke on "Cost-Benefit Analysis of Regulatory Actions" to the members of the National Advisory Food and Drug Committee (NAFDC) and made it clear that only during that year had FDA started to apply cost-benefit techniques. In response to the following

---

81. William Wardell, "The Development and Allocation of Medical Care Resources: Administrative Aspects," speech, World Medical Assembly Symposium, Tokyo, October 8, 1975, mimeo, p. 5.

remark of a staff member, that "I think it might be useful to mention how many economists we (FDA) now have. How many do we have?[*sic*]" Barkdoll replied: "Well, we really have one. (laughter)"[82]

An in-depth inflation impact statement is now required of any proposed new regulation which, after being pre-screened in five specified areas for any potential inflationary impact, then is evaluated as to whether it is likely to have an overall inflationary impact on the economy. It is this Executive Order and the Sunshine Acts which have forced FDA to use cost-benefit analysis. Barkdoll stated that FDA as of November 20, 1975, had pre-screened all proposed regulations for potential inflationary impact and then "approximately 25 evaluations of specific proposals" were made in order to explain why these proposed regulations would not have a major inflationary impact in terms of the Executive Order's criteria. Barkdoll also stated that FDA in order to do the screening obtains all the secondary data which it can, assumes the worst case resulting from the proposed regulation, and costs it out. This creates delay. In all twenty-five preliminary inflation analyses made prior to November 20, 1975, FDA had "not found one which exceeds any of the five"[83] criteria and, therefore, no in-depth inflation impact statement to that date had been prepared.[84]

However, FDA six months later announced its first in-depth inflation impact analysis and judged that "a major inflation impact" would result from banning furazolidone (Nitrofuran) in food-producing animals. The proposed ban summarizes that the anticipated impact would be to reduce poultry production, including broilers, turkey, and eggs, from 2 percent in the first year of the ban up to 20 percent in later years, depending on suppliers' reactions; and to reduce similarly swine production from 0 percent in the first year to 5 percent in later years. The higher estimates, applicable to later years, depend on the rates of increase in diseases which will occur when this antibacterial is banned from the feed of the animals. "The per-capita cost annual increases are equivalent to an aggregate ranging from $291 million to $2.635 billion." The benefit of "the elimination of any risk of any cancer associated with the consumption, via the edible tissues" of animals ingesting furazolidone was judged to outweigh the costs.[85]

Barkdoll had elaborated at the NAFDC November 1976 meeting that in screening, "you just worry about costs," but if forced into doing an in-depth inflation impact statement, then "you must discuss both benefits and

---
82. U.S. FDA, NAFDC *Transcript,* November 20, 1975, p. 89.
83. Ibid., p. 69.
84. Ibid.
85. Federal Register, May 13, 1976, p. 19906.

costs" and "now sometimes we do the cost-benefit not because it's required, but because that's the way the decision will be made."[86] It is interesting to me as an economist that it apparently took that long for the planning and evaluation arm of the FDA to realize that in decision making, all costs should be related to all benefits because it is the net benefits, not only adverse effects, which are most important to the decision. Cost-benefit analysis, not merely an inflation impact statement, is broader than a biological risk-benefit analysis. It also offers an opportunity to compare by a single measure, the dollar costs and benefits. The summary of FDA's first inflation impact statement as it appeared in the *Federal Register* does not mention a dollar value of anticipated benefits. It is possible that the in-depth analysis on file with the FDA hearing clerk, does. To measure the anticipated benefits there would have to be some biological data on the probability of cancer occurring in the population at risk from eating the poultry (including eggs, broilers, turkey) and the pork products. Since "scientists using radioactive tracers and other new methods have been finding ever smaller traces of carcinogens in foods. . .,"[87] as low as 0.1 part per billion, and since testing of carcinogens usually involve exceedingly high amounts of the suspected carcinogen ingested by animals, such data would have been useful to the reader of only the summary.

To some degree, FDA has been forced to use a form of cost-benefit analysis in order to protect its own interests. A new Economic Analysis Group of the FDA was established in the third quarter of the fiscal year 1975 "to provide support in the analysis of economic factors and economic impact of FDA regulatory decisions. It will provide initial guidance in the preparation of Inflation Impact Statements (as directed by the President's Executive Order) and other economic analyses of significant Agency issues."[88]

Commissioner Schmidt has expressed concern about the effect on food supplies and thus prices if antibacterials used in feed of small animals and in feed (DES) of large animals are banned in the United States. These raise a basic economic question which requires not only economic analysis but also biological data, even if the latter cannot be quantified to help resolve what is a value judgment. Recently Commissioner Schmidt described his thinking about the difficult problem of reaching a decision when all data are not available, and if available, are not quantifiable:

> . . . we are in the business of balancing benefit and risk. And it comes down ultimately to a judgment. One of the reasons that we are trying to

---

86. U.S. FDA, NAFDC *Transcript,* op. cit., p. 69.
87. Campbell, op. cit., p. 5.
88. U.S. FDA *Quarterly Activities Report,* Third Quarter, Fiscal Year 1975, p. 12.

open up the agency, that we are using and will continue to use advisory committees, that we are seeking expert help, is so that we can have the best possible judgment. Each case is so different. The judgment must be tailored to the diseases, to the conditions, to the type of side effects, to the amount of suffering that's involved, and so on.[89]

Physicians' major objections to use of an economic approach and their disdain for "economists" derive from the attempts by economists to place a dollar value on life and loss of limb. This is held to be proof of economists' lack of reverence for life and a display of their crassness, which automatically places the profession of economists below that of physicians—at least from a humanistic point of view. The economist's concern is to estimate the economic benefits derived from the maintenance and prolongation of life, and also the benefits which occur when individuals' abilities to enjoy a higher level of quality of life are increased, as when a drug enables them to work while otherwise disease would prevent this level of activity. This is also a humanistic concern. Prolongation of life is not the only benefit which a drug may confer. Placing a dollar value on the net benefit is a convenient method of measuring humanistic concern and is the best measure now available.

Economists, and also physicians, recognize that everyone must ultimately die. Risk-benefit ratios are estimated for different options to attain a given goal or to evaluate a range of goals from which a decision is to be made. If the data used involves risk of death and/or averting death, an assumed valuation of life is implied although it is not usually stated as such.

The peculiar arrogance which does not accept that other than medically trained professionals have the competence to weigh the relative value of conflicting data often surfaced during NADC meetings. There was no lawyer, and I was the only economist on the NADC during the three-year period in which I served. Most of the "expert science" FDA committees did not have a biostatistician.[90]

Among the real experts on a given drug are the company scientists who have developed the drug which may be their own brainchild; therefore, they have a conflict of interest. But, most academic physicians and research scientists who, with their institutions, receive sizeable federal grants also have conflicts of interest. Greater use of biostatisticians and other professionally trained scientists might make selection of an unbiased, "expert" committee easier. Some streamlining of the long IND-NDA approval process could

---

89. Alexander Schmidt in *Reforming Federal Drug Regulation,* "Round Table," February 23, 1976 (Washington, D.C.: AEI, 1976), pp. 26, 27.
90. The Drug Experience Advisory Committee had an epidemiologist, and at least one exception was the Pulmonary-Allergy and Clinical Immunology Advisory Committee.

possibly be attained by accepting company expertise, at least in the initial phases of investigation when the risk of unknown hazards of new drugs to humans is small. Any bias could then be offset by exposing that expertise during the later phases of drug testing to a combination of the adversary procedure and biostatistician, research, and clinical physician reviews.

The Public Interest

At times throughout this study, references have been made to the "public interest" in the government regulation of drugs. It has been assumed, but without being stated specifically that assurance of a degree of drug safety is in the public interest and, therefore, this alone is a sound basis for government regulation of the marketing of drugs.

Safety and Efficacy

Whether "safety" can be logically separated from the second criterion "efficacy" added by the 1962 amendments appears to be debatable. No drug which confers a benefit is completely safe and has zero risk. Therefore, safety is not an absolute factor when it is applied to drugs. The law gives a negative mandate to FDA: to protect the public from harm. But all drugs may harm. Complete safety is impossible to attain. What is probably acceptable to the public are those drugs with no close substitutes which, when appropriately used, create benefits that in total outweigh the rare incidence of a serious side effect. The problem involves an assessment of the value of a life and the reader is referred to my writing elsewhere on this subject for a brief discussion and short bibliography.[91]

Efficacy also is not an absolute factor when applied to drugs, but connotes degrees of benefit. Evaluation of the risk and the benefit of a drug assesses safety against efficacy and it is this approach which FDA uses. For that reason I believe that the British policy initiated in 1965 by their Committee on Safety of Drugs and reaffirmed by their new Committee on Safety of Medicines in its first report for the calendar year 1971, under the new British statutory control of the Medicines Acts 1968 and 1971, is the more desirable approach from the point of view of the public interest. Therefore, the relative Section 6.2 of that report, issued in September 1972, is quoted at length as follows:

The Committee believed that the main purpose of the Act was to

---

91. Campbell, op. cit., pp. 19-21.

provide a safeguard against indiscriminate promotion of dangerously toxic medicines or medicines of inadequate quality, but that it had never been intended that it should be used to deny to the public a large number of products which presented no hazard. The Committee believed that in the case of herbal, homeopathic and other unorthodox remedies it would be possible to ensure, for example by labelling requirements, that the public were aware that they had been considered so far as effectiveness was concerned, in terms of their own particular theory of medicine. For all other medicinal products the Committee considered that it was important that the public should not be misled by claims which were unsubstantiated [*sic*]. It was agreed accordingly to adhere to the policy, originally stated by the Committee on Safety of Drugs in 1965, that the Committee must consistently consider efficacy in relation to safety. If a medicine not known to be effective were recommended for the treatment of a serious illness for which there was already a satisfactory treatment, this would constitute an unacceptable risk to the patient. Similarly if a medicine were likely to be quite ineffective in the treatment of any disease for which it was recommended and yet carried the slightest risk to the patient, the Committee would regard it as unsafe for use as recommended.[92]

If this interpretation of efficacy were accepted by U.S. law, and if it were coupled with a more rigorous postmarket review of drugs and some streamlining of IND and NDA procedures, then the delay which the United States has been experiencing in availability of new, effective drugs would be lessened. Dr. Zubrod's testimony September 1974, in respect to drugs effective against cancer cited earlier, is clear indication that even when the existing alternative drugs are not efficacious and the disease is terminal our regulatory system is not an ideal one, even when there is positive government support as by the Cancer Institute. It is likely to be a less ideal system for approval of drugs for diseases of lesser seriousness.

The importance of labelling and more effective communication to the public, not only to the physician, also should be emphasized, especially if a less rigorous standard for efficacy is used. Even if the same standards are upheld, the area of communication to the public needs considerable improvement in addition to the changes recently implemented by FDA.

The British report of September 1972 comments from the British regulatory point of view on FDA's November 1970 list of 369 drugs for which FDA accepted the classification by the National Academy of Sciences and National Research Council's review as "dangerous and ineffective." Ninety products on

---

92. United Kingdom, Committee on Safety of Medicines, *Annual Report for the Year Ended 31st December, 1971* (London: Her Majesty's Stationery Office, SB N 11 3203004, September 1972), pp. 9, 10.

this list were known to the Committee on Safety of Medicines to be available in Great Britain either as "identical or very similar to products in the FDA list."[93]

> When considering these products the Committee noted that in many cases the FDA withdrawal notices were issued because there was not considered to be substantial evidence that the products were effective. The Committee, however, in accordance with its terms of reference, considers the efficacy of drugs only in relation to their safety.
>
> On the evidence available to it about the products included in the list and on sale in the United Kingdom the Committee concluded that those products on sale directly to the public did not present any hazards serious enough to justify their withdrawal from the market, and that those which were available only on prescription presented no special risk not already well documented and known to the medical and pharmaceutical professions.[94]

The United Kingdom is a smaller country than ours, but does have, today, a diversified population. The British government is more willing to rely on the common sense of the physician/patient consumer, once informed, than we are. They have made mistakes, but our system also makes mistakes. There is need for an in-depth study of the benefits and costs of the present United States regulatory system of drugs.

Research on Drugs

Has the regulatory system only delayed use of more effective therapeutic drugs than were in existence in the United States in recent years, or is it also driving abroad the research and development of new drugs by U.S. pharmaceutical companies? The latter, if true, is lessening employment and pushing the first marketing of new drugs developed by American companies outside the United States.

The fifteen largest U.S.-owned drug companies, accounting for about 80 percent of U.S. research and development in the pharmaceutical industry, have been during the last five years increasingly doing research abroad, especially clinical studies which test their new chemical entities (NCEs) in man.[95] IND applications submitted annually for new chemical entities in the

---

93. Ibid.
94. Ibid., pp. 8, 9.
95. Louis Lasagna and William Wardell, "The Rate of New Drug Discovery," in *Drug Development and Marketing,* edited by Robert Helms (Washington, D.C.: AEI, 1975), p. 157. NCE "defined as a compound a molecular structure, not previously tested in man, excluding new salts, vaccines and diagnostic agents."

years 1971-73 were only one-half (thirty-seven per year) than what they had been during 1963-65 when they averaged seventy-four per year.[96] The average (mean) time required for clinical study and approval of NDAs has increased from 2.5 years in 1966 to 6.6 years in 1973.[97]

Although the number of active NCE-INDs has steadily increased, the percent of NDAs or approvals has fallen to less than 1 percent of all NCE-IND filings since 1968, and to an average of 4.5 percent of all such filings from 1963 through April 1974.[98]

The worldwide decline in the number of NCEs gives some credence to the theory that "the easy nuts have been cracked;" but the drastic change by U.S. companies from doing early drug research on humans in the United States to doing it abroad offers an alternative explanation as does the fact that other countries have also been increasing their regulatory requirements. It is possible that worldwide regulation is depressing creative innovation. It is also possible that U.S. basic research is being exploited for new drugs abroad, but before such a conclusion can be reached more data are needed.

Worldwide, there are no effective drugs for many common diseases for which large markets offer sales and profits, and breakthroughs in these areas should be forthcoming soon.

> . . . most of the basic knowledge that the industry has been working on has been produced by research in the basic sciences; therefore it is to assessments of basic research that we must turn to examine whether the hypothesis is based on correct premises. . . .
>
> Basic knowledge about disease and therapeutics is increasing at an exponential rate, as is apparent to any scientist who attends scientific meetings and reads the literature. The National Institutes of Health have channeled vast funds into basic biomedical research over the past 15 years; these now exceed over a billion dollars per year, and research productivity, as evidenced by the rate of scientific advance would appear to be increasing rather than decreasing, as powerful new research techniques continue to be developed.

The most up-to-date and prestigious assessment of this situation is available from the President's Biomedical Research Panel, which reported in April, 1976.

The findings of the President's Biomedical Research Panel suggest the opposite of the "knowledge depletion" hypothesis. In the report of the Overview Cluster, under the heading "The Future Impact of Biomedical Science," the Report notes:

---

96. Ibid., p. 158.
97. Ibid., p. 160.
98. Ibid., p. 161.

Human beings have within reach the capacity to control or prevent human disease. Although this may seem an overly optimistic forecast, it is, in fact a realistic, practical appraisal of the long-term future. The historical record of accomplishment to date, having plainly established that some of the most lethal, complex, and previously baffling human diseases can be eliminated (or at least held in check), seems to us a warrant for optimism. Perhaps it would be prudent and realistic to insert a qualifying phrase: the capacity to *learn how* to control or prevent human disease is within reach.

There do not appear to be any impenetrable, incomprehensible diseases. This, in itself, represents the major advance for biomedical science, and it is a change which has occurred only within the past 25 years.

Under the heading, "The Relation of Industry and University Science," the Overview Cluster states:

> At the current pace of scientific progress, especially in such fields as neurobiology, psychopharmacology, and immunopharmacology, it can be predicted that opportunities will steadily increase for the development of entirely new classes of drugs.[99]

Rare Diseases

It is also in the public interest for government not to compete in those areas where the economic incentives to private industry are great enough that no additional stimulus is needed. FDA could, from a political and logical point of view, be given the mandate to stimulate research for drugs for rare disease, for example by subsidizing such research through its own grants and the grants jointly awarded with the National Institutes of Health (NIH). A strict application of cost-benefit analysis may not support government expenditures for research to alleviate or cure rare disease, because so few persons may benefit and the costs of the research may be higher than the total benefits. The valuation of the benefits depend on the assumed valuation of life (or the improved quality of living) which involves different discount rates and other complications which to explain here would distract from the main line of thought of this monograph. However, it is difficult to predict what the additional costs of research may be to discover therapeutic drugs for rare diseases. Effective therapeutic drugs for some rare diseases have been

---

99. William Wardell, "Regulation and Pharmaceutical Innovation: A Review of the Relationship Between Government Regulation Aimed at Protecting Health and Human Safety, and Innovation Leading to Medically Useful Drugs," written for the National Science Foundation, June 1976, mimeo, pp. 64, 65.

developed relatively inexpensively by pharmaceutical companies. Such drugs often have been a serendipitous side-effect of research on other drugs which are anticipated to be profitable drugs because they are aimed at alleviation or cure of common diseases and therefore have promise of large sales.

Second uses of marketed drugs have also been a source of therapeutic gains for the less common diseases and it is an approach which government should not discourage. FDA in August 1972, by publishing a notice in the *Federal Register,* attempted to improve the situation.[100] Dr. Finkel writes that the notice's "primary purpose . . . was to clarify the legal status of the package insert." Among other items, the package insert specifies the indication for which a marketed drug is labelled. The notice also outlined "the steps that FDA could take to assure that package inserts are current with scientific knowledge. These include: (1) requests for manufacturers to gather data on new uses or (2) independent assessments by the FDA and its advisors that adequate information exists in the literature to approve the new uses and to provide appropriate directions for use."[101] Despite FDA's acknowledgement that physicians may legally prescribe drugs for other than the labelled indication, the labelling of drugs as therapy for a specific diagnosis, in the current unfortunate climate of ever ready malpractice suits, makes physicians wary of using drugs for a diagnosis not indicated by the mandated labelling and, therefore, this may diminish the intuitive, serendipitous discovery of new uses for old drugs.

Safe but Ineffective Drugs

From an economist's point of view, the use of highly trained manpower, short in supply within FDA, to prepare a case against the apparently increasing numbers of persons using non-effective, but safe drugs appears to be a misallocation of scarce resources which might be better used in processing applications for probably effective drugs.

If full information is given to the public as well as to the physician or pharmacist about an ineffective but safe drug, then the decision of whether or not to use that drug, it might be argued, should be the consumer's—defined as the patient/physician. If all patient-physician relationships were the ideal confidential type, no harm might occur. Unfortunately, however, there are some physicians who would, as some illegally do today, use their personal influence to lead terminally ill patients away from use of acceptable, more

---

100. *Federal Register,* August 17, 1972, p. 16503.
101. Marion Finkel, "The Benefit/Risk Ratio of New Drug Regulation in the United States," *The Internist,* March 1974, p. 15.

effective but probably more risky, drugs and/or other treatment. It is possible that this would increase the number of physicians acting in this fashion.

Better continuing education of physicians, better self-policing of the profession, and more understanding by all physicians of those patients who do not wish to continue or even begin what they believe is ineffective and demeaning treatment are also needed. Medicine is an art as well as a science and placebos are effective; otherwise why are controlled studies required?

Physicians who currently make a profit from the illegal sales of such drugs which are harmless *per se*, but which may be judged harmful in that they substitute for more effective treatment, would lose that profit if the drugs could be legally sold. What the trade-offs are between, on the one hand, removing government regulation of a paternalistic nature in this very limited area and, on the other hand, increasing the time involved in the processing of INDs and NDAs, I do not have the facts to evaluate. However, Dr. Zubrod's testimony as to the length of delay in approval of effective drugs for cancer indicates that there is some trade-off.

To classify harmless drugs legally with addictive drugs, such as heroin, ensures that some persons will make a profit from their sale. The British approach may be better and at least it should be considered in debate.

Cost-Benefit Analysis and Decision Making on Drugs

The thought processes of the individual who makes public policy decisions, whether in science or other areas, may be more structured by requiring use of cost-benefit analysis techniques, which are especially useful for national resource allocation decisions.

One academic research physician who has been an investigator of new drugs and done considerable work on drug lag, including drug case histories, recently concluded that "My own experience suggests that the differences [in decision making] lie with individual monitors within the FDA, and with their personal standards and philosophy."[102] This comment seems to be borne out in part by the 906 pages of the detailed *Commissioner's Report. . .1975* by Alexander Schmidt, which explores in detail the previously mentioned allegations, by eleven of FDA's lower level physicians, of "harassment" by higher level FDA officials.

If actual cost-benefit analysis rather than risk-benefit analysis had been

---

102. Louis Lasagna, "Bureaucratic Controls Will Stifle Both Industry and Intelligent Medical Practice," in *Controversy in Internal Medicine,* vol. 2, edited by F.J. Ingelfinger et al. (Philadelphia: Saunders, 1974), p. 77.

routinely used in policy decisions by FDA, then some of the actions detailed in the *Commissioner's Report. . .1975* would not have occurred; as, for example, the discontinuation by Squibb Co. of their IND (Number 6032), originally submitted August 8, 1969. This was an application to conduct "a double-blind placebo controlled study of whether chronic administration of 5-grain aspirin (four times daily for two years) would affect the myocardial infarction rate and mortality of 400 post-myocardial infarct patients."[103] Squibb finally gave up this research because the company felt that it literally could not meet the rules being imposed by the FDA monitors, such as to submit "all known reports on aspirin." They felt that this was excessive for an over-the-counter drug marketed in the United States since 1899. An FDA physician was able to force discontinuance of this IND in 1970.[104] I find Commissioner Schmidt's comment on the matter to be laudable insofar as it goes.

> Dr. Nestor sought to apply rigidly the requirements of the IND regulations in a situation where such application seemed unreasonable to his colleagues and supervisors. It is difficult to criticize someone who goes by the literal word of FDA's rules, yet one must recognize that sometimes the results can be counterproductive to the public health, and even foolish. The investigators under this protocol could have lawfully carried out their study, without filing an IND, by using aspirin available in any over the counter package. The desire to utilize aspirin with a standardized quality obtained directly from a manufacturer was what necessitated a submission to FDA. Further, the study was to gain important knowledge relating to the use of aspirin in conjunction with serious heart disease, not to develop a unique product for marketing; thus the incentive to mislead the FDA was nil. (If the study did indicate a new use for aspirin, it would be of very limited commercial value to the sponsor, considering the great competition in the OTC aspirin market.) Treating this IND as though aspirin were a novel entity for which a thorough preclinical workup was necessary, resulted in termination of the study. I find that Dr. Nestor's mechanical approach to this IND reflected an adversarial [sic] concept of the FDA's role in drug studies. This concept is wholly inappropriate to the Agency's function and inconsistent with good science which encourages skepticism and questioning but not dogmation [sic] or hostility.[105]

But an economist and an epidemiologist would go further than Commissioner Schmidt. Many persons with rheumatoid arthritis have taken far more than four 5-grain aspirin daily (a common dosage is eight 5-grain aspirin daily) over long periods of time. The vital statistics section of NIH has data on

---

103. Schmidt, *Commissioner's Report. . .1975,* mimeo, p. 183.
104. Ibid., p. 186.
105. Ibid., pp. 186-87.

deaths in 1955 by multiple diagnoses which would cover those years before the greater usage of different drugs became common for treatment of this disease. A computer cross-tabulation using the data tapes of the mortality rate from myocardial infarction of persons with rheumatoid arthritis from these data might, because of the large numbers of persons involved, be very revealing even if the aspirin dosage were not standardized and no controls were involved. It is possible by now that a retrospective study, utilizing sophisticated statistical techniques which would indicate the confidence limits, is being done along these lines. A very brief search of recent literature has turned up several articles relating aspirin and coronary heart disease, but there appears to be no firm conclusive relationship, partly because each study seems to have some statistical fault—the retrospective ones especially not using a standard dosage.[106] One retrospective study of sixty-two patients who died during the period 1950-72, but with the more precise definition of myocardial infarction and with some apparent control over aspirin dosage, states that although "data show a significant reduction in the morbidity and mortality of MI [myocardial infarction] in the group of patients with rheumatoid arthritis," the study concludes that "the data do not permit the conclusion that this drug [aspirin] prevented MI in our patients with RA [rheumatoid arthritis]. Only controlled prospective studies can determine the efficacy of this or any other agent in the prevention of MI. However, we have shown that, for whatever reason, the incidence of MI is significantly reduced in at least some patients with RA. . . ."[107]

Today a $16 million study, funded by the NIH involving 4,200 patients, is being conducted by Rush Presbyterian-St. Luke Medical Center, Chicago, to test whether aspirin does decrease risk of a second heart attack.[108] Furthermore, several other international studies of aspirin for this same purpose are already beginning to show beneficial results on heart attack and mortality.

To turn down prospective, controlled double-blind clinical studies of good design which have not been previously done and where the disease, MI, is a major cause of death is in Dr. Schmidt's words "foolish" and not in the public

---

106. See, for example, E. Culyer Hammond and Lawrence Garfinkel, "Aspirin and Coronary Heart Disease: Findings of a Prospective Study," *British Medical Journal*, 1975, vol. 2, pp. 269-71, and especially their "Discussion on two retrospective studies of the Boston Collaborative Drug Surveillance Group." The latter's "results seemed to indicate that the relative risk of acute myocardial infarction is about one-fifth as high (first study) or about half as high (second study) in regular aspirin users as in other people." p. 271.
107. Richard Davis and Edgar Engleman, "Incidence of Myocardial Infarction in Patients with Rheumatoid Arthritis," *Arthritis and Rheumatism*, vol. 17, no. 5, September-October 1974, pp. 531, 532.
108. *Wall Street Journal*, June 9, 1976, p. 1.

interest. If cost-benefit analysis were added to the rules of procedure, literal interpretation of this nature might be avoided in the future. A four to six-year or longer delay in obtaining an answer as apparently has occurred in this instance, and in a similar delay in medical advice acting on the data, probably has cost millions of dollars of gross national product—if aspirin is, as it appears to be, effective in preventing myocardial infarction, sudden death, and even stroke. Failure to approach this from a humanistic point of view—to use a favorite phrase of some physicians—is, of course, obvious.

In April 1975, FDA issued its "Program Management System" (PMS) Blue Book to serve as guidelines for FDA managers. It states:

Project priorities are rated with respect to three criteria:

> RISK: The real loss or injury experienced by the public, i.e., the remaining problem or hazard to be eliminated.
>
> SENSITIVITY: Intensity of interest as expressed by consumers, Congress, the Administration and industry. High sensitivity is typically engendered by high consumer vulnerability and lack of product substitutes.
>
> POTENTIAL EFFECTIVENESS: The expected impact of additional resources on risk reduction.[109]

The emphasis of the three criteria is on risks and not on benefits, and *risk* is not equivalent to *cost* in the sense in which an economist uses the word. The PMS guidelines used by FDA do not follow the customary cost-benefit analysis approach: to estimate a net benefit for a range of options to solve a particular problem.

The separating out of "sensitivity," which covers "public and political perception. . .," indicates that this criterion is also important in decision making by the top echelon of FDA on planning, budgeting, and evaluation.[110]

Concern over the integration of national science policy with socio-economic policy has been expressed in several recent government reports. For example, a recent *Congressional Joint Economic Committee Report*, known as the *Gilpin Report* (written by Professor Robert Gilpin of Princeton University) concludes:

> "The overall recommendation of this report is that technology policy must be coupled with socio-economic policy. At all levels of policymaking and across the broad spectrum of government activities, technological options and user-needs (or market-demand) must be brought

---

109. U.S. HEW, FDA, *FY 1976 PMS Blue Book,* April 1975, mimeo, p. 2.
110. Ibid., Appendix 1, p. 181.

together and integrated in policymaking. Such a recommendation seems self-evident and easy to accomplish. In fact, the coupling of these two aspects of government policy is too seldom achieved. While in theory it is easy to do, in practice it is exceptionally difficult because of institutional commitments and lack of sufficient knowledge.[111]

This report states further:

> Undoubtedly the most critical and least appreciated aspect of technological innovation is the problem of uncertainty. As we have seen, technical and economic uncertainty surrounds all innovation and cannot be completely eliminated, though it can be reduced by better management methods, technological assessment, and so forth.[112]

To aid in the goal of integrating scientific and socio-economic national policy, cost-benefit analysis can be most helpful. The public interest requires that creative technology, especially in the health sector, not be hampered by excessive government regulation.

To limit the use of economists within FDA to only the "Economic Analysis Group" and to work only on inflation impact statements and the economic effect of proposed regulations would underutilize their potential to work in the interest of public health. Interdisciplinary research at the early stages of initial design of drug studies is needed. In FDA, as in the Environmental Protection Agency, all persons involved in policy decisions would make better decisions if they were acquainted with cost-benefit analysis so that they weigh all the costs; and "all" is defined to include the loss of potential benefits from a given course of action. Emphasis on only biological risk is too costly to the public's true interest.

That a drug lag probably still exists in the United States in some therapeutic areas was implied by Commissioner Schmidt in a debate, February 23, 1976, as follows:

> Beclomethasone, the asthma drug that Lou [Lasagna] mentioned, was developed overseas. It was introduced in England many years before it came here—which was just a couple of years ago—as an application to the FDA. The application was deficient. We have been working as quickly as we can to bring that drug into the marketplace in this country, when our requirements are satisfied. But we cannot approve a drug for which we don't have an application.
>
> So the drug lag has to be analyzed. It has to be broken down. I think Lou has said that there has never been a real drug lag in antibiotics or in

---

111. Robert Gilpin, *Technology, Economic and International Competitiveness* (a report), July 9, 1975, p. 65.
112. Ibid., p. 67.

certain other drugs; cardiovascular drugs have, I think, been the big problem that people point to.[113]

Although the NADC's advice was purely advisory and did not have to be taken—and sometimes was not—by the commissioner, the committee did serve not only as a "sounding board" and "window dressing" for some decisions made by the commissioner, but acted to prevent a delay by FDA in considering seriously the Dripps Committee's charges of a drug lag in the United States. The NADC as such was phased out when its remaining members were merged with the remaining members of the National Advisory Food Committee and National Advisory Veterinary Committee to form the new NAFDC, which first met March 27, 1975.

To summarize, I quote the last sentence of the National Science Foundations report, *Chemicals and Health:* "Finally, regardless of the type of review and analysis mechanisms chosen, the Panel finds great virtue in explicit explanation to the public as to how decisions are arrived at, what assumptions are included and what information is used."[114]

This monograph is an attempt to add to the type of background literature referred to above as to how public policy decision making takes place, and also to stimulate debate about the complex problems involved in regulation of drugs by the government.

---

113. Schmidt in *Reforming Federal Drug Regulation*, op. cit., pp. 4, 5.
114. U.S. NSF, *Chemicals and Health*, Report of the Panel on Chemicals and Health of the President's Science Advisory Committee, September 1973, p. 139.

Selected Bibliography

Books

Campbell, Rita Ricardo. *Food Safety Regulation: A Study of the Use and Limitations of Cost-Benefit Analysis.* AEI-Hoover Policy Studies, no. 12. Washington, D.C.: American Enterprise Institute/Hoover Institution Press, August 1974. See the Selected Bibliography, pp. 55-59, which lists several background books and articles that are not repeated in this bibliography.

Cooper, Joseph, ed. *The Philosophy of Evidence: Philosophy and Technology of Drug Assessment,* vol. 3. Washington, D.C.: Interdisciplinary Communications, Inc., 1972.

———. *Regulation, Economics and Pharmaceutical Innovation.* Proceedings of the second seminar on Pharmaceutical Public Policy Issues. Washington, D.C.: American University, 1973.

Decision Making for Regulating Chemicals in the Environment (a report). Washington, D.C.: National Academy of Sciences, 1975. See especially chapter 8, "Information on Benefits."

Helms, Robert B., ed. *Drug Development and Marketing.* Washington, D.C.: AEI, 1975.

How Safe Is Safe? The Design of Policy on Drugs and Food Additives. Washington, D.C.: National Academy of Sciences, 1974.

Landau, Richard, ed. *Regulating New Drugs.* Chicago: University of Chicago Press, 1973.

Peltzman, Sam. *Regulation of Pharmaceutical Innovation.* Washington, D.C.: AEI, June 1974.

Reforming Federal Drug Regulation. "Round Table," February 23, 1976. Washington, D.C.: AEI, 1976.

Taylor, David, ed. *Benefits and Risks in Medical Care.* Proceedings of a symposium held in London, March 1974. London: Office of Health Economics, 1974.

Wardell, William, and Lasagna, Louis. *Regulation and Drug Development.* Washington, D.C.: AEI, July 1975.

Articles, Papers, and Government Publications

Davis, Richard F., and Engleman, Edgar G. "Incidence of Myocardial Infarction in Patients with Rheumatoid Arthritis." *Arthritis and Rheumatism,* vol. 17, no. 5, September-October, 1974, pp. 527-33.

De Haen, Paul. "New Drugs in Europe." *New York State Journal of Medicine,* March 15, 1973, pp. 777-80.

Dukes, M.N.G. "Law, Medicines and the Doctor: A Critical Look at Drug Regulation." *Current Medical Research and Opinion,* vol. 1, no. 10, 1973, pp. 612-28.

Edwards, Charles. "The Role of Government and FDA Regulation in Drug R&D." *Research Management,* March 1974, pp. 21-23.

Finkel, Marion. "The Benefit/Risk Ratio of New Drug Regulation in the United States." *The Internist,* March 1974, pp. 10-15.

Gilpin, Robert. *Technology, Economic and International Competitiveness.* A report for U.S. Congress, Joint Economic Committee. Washington, D.C.: Government Printing Office, July 1975.

Greenberg, David. "FDA: Poor Marks for Its Self-Investigation." *New England Journal of Medicine,* vol. 294, no. 26, pp. 1465-66.

Hammond, E. Culyer, and Garfinkel, Lawrence. "Aspirin and Coronary Heart Disease: Findings of a Prospective Study." *British Medical Journal,* 1975, no. 2, pp. 269-71.

Hollister, Leo. "The FDA Ten Years After the Kefauver-Harris Amendment." *Perspectives in Biology and Medicine,* winter 1974, pp. 242-49.

Lasagna, Louis. "Bureaucratic Controls Will Stifle Both Industry and Intelligent Medical Practice." In *Controversy in Internal Medicine,* vol. 2, edited by F.J. Ingelfinger et al. Philadelphia: Saunders, 1974, pp. 74-80.

Lasagna, Louis and Wardell, William. "The Rate of New Drug Discovery." in *Drug Development and Marketing,* edited by Robert Helms. Washington, D.C.: AEI, 1975, pp. 155-81.

Ley, Herbert. "Federal Regulation Is Essential to Protect the Patient." In *Controversy in Internal Medicine,* vol. 2, edited by F.J. Ingelfinger et al. Philadelphia: Saunders, 1974, pp. 67-73.

Lublin, Joan. "Uncommon Pill? Aspirin Might Help Heart Attacks." *Wall Street Journal,* June 9, 1976, pp. 1, 22.

McGuire, Thomas, et. al. "An Evaluation of Consumer Protection Legislation: The 1962 Amendments: A Comment." *Journal of Political Economy,* vol. 83, no. 31, 1975, pp. 655-59.

Peltzman, Sam. "An Evaluation of Consumer Protection Legislation: The 1962 Drug Amendments: A Reply." *Journal of Political Economy,* vol. 83, no. 3, 1975, pp. 663-67.

Reis-Arndt, E., and Elvers, D. "Results of Pharma Research: New Pharmaceutical Agents 1961-1970." In *Drugs Made in Germany,* vol. 5, no. 3, Ingelheim, West Germany: C.H. Boehringer Sohn, 1972, pp. 134-40.

Sarett, Lewis. "FDA Regulations and Their Influence on Future R & D." *Research Management,* March 1974, p. 18-20.

Simmons, Henry. "Prescription Drugs and American Patients." *FDA Consumer,* November 1973.

United Kingdom, Committee on Safety of Medicines. *Annual Report for the Year Ended 31st December, 1971.* London: Her Majesty's Stationery Office, SB N 11 3203004, September 1972.

U.S. Federal Register. Washington, D.C.: Government Printing Office. August 17, 1972, p. 16503; September 6, 1973, pp. 24220-22; April 9, 1975, pp. 16053-57; May 13, 1976, p. 19906.

U.S. Food and Drug Administration. *Public Advisory Committees: Authority, Structure, Functions, Members.* Washington, D.C.: Government Printing Office, 1974 ed. and 1975 ed.

———. *Quarterly Activities Report,* Fourth Quarter, Fiscal Year 1975. Washington, D.C.: Government Printing Office 896-202.

U.S. House of Representatives, Committee on Appropriations, Subcommittee on Agriculture-Environmental and Consumer Protection, *Appropriations for 1975: Hearings,* Part 8, May 6, 1974, FDA "Study of the Delaney Clause and Other Anti-cancer Clauses." Washington, D.C.: Government Printing Office.

U.S. House of Representatives, Committee on Government Operations. *Use of Advisory Committees by the Food and Drug Administration.* 11th Report. January 26, 1976. House Report 94-787.

U.S. National Science Foundation, *Chemicals and Health.* Report of the Panel on Chemicals and Health of the President's Science Advisory Committee. Washington, D.C.: Government Printing Office, September 1973.

Wardell, William M. "The Assessment of the Benefits, Risks and Costs of Medical Progress." In *Benefits and Risks in Medical Care,* edited by David Taylor. London: Office of Health Economics, 1974, pp. 93-104.

———. "British Usage and American Awareness of Some New Therapeutic Drugs." *Clinical Pharmacology and Therapeutics,* vol. 14, 1973, pp. 1022-34.

———. "Fluroxene and the Penicillin Lesson." *Anesthesiology,* vol. 38, no. 4, April 1973, pp. 309 ff.

———. "Introduction of New Therapeutic Drugs in the United States and Great Britain: An International Comparison." *Clinical Pharmacology and Therapeutics,* vol. 14, 1973, pp. 773-90.

———. "Therapeutic Implications of the Drug Lag." *Clinical Pharmacology and Therapeutics,* vol. 15, 1974, pp. 73-96.

Zubrod, C. Gordon. Statement in U.S. Senate, Select Committee on Small Business, Subcommittee on Monopoly. In *Hearings on Competitive Problems in the Drug Industry.* Washington, D.C.: Government Printing Office, 1973, part 23, pp. 9672-81.

Unpublished Material

Azarnoff, Daniel. Statement in U.S. Senate, Select Committee on Small Business, Subcommittee on Monopoly, February 6, 1973. Mimeographed.

"The Citizen and the Expert." The Academy Forum (proceedings). January 20, 1976. Washington, D.C.: National Academy of Sciences. Mimeographed.

Cooper, Joseph. "The Control of Medical Innovation and Prescribing by the FDA." Speech given at the annual meeting of the American Association for the Advancement of Science, New York, January 27, 1975. Mimeographed.

Crout, Richard. Remarks to the U.S. Department of Health, Education, and Welfare, Review Panel on New Drug Regulation, April 19, 1976. Unofficial thermographic copy of a transcript from a non-professionally recorded tape.

———. Statement in U.S. Senate, Joint Hearings: Committee on Labor and Public Welfare—Subcommittee on Health, and Committee on Judiciary—Subcommittee on Administration Practice and Procedure, September 27, 1974. Mimeographed transcript. Part of a panel debate on drug lag with Dr. William Wardell, Dr. John Oates, Dr. Richard Crout, and Dr. Thomas Chalmers.

Dripps, Robert. Statement, National Advisory Drug Committee meeting, November 30, 1972. Mimeographed.

Edwards, Charles. "Meeting New Challenges." Speech before the Food and Drug Law Institute, Washington, D.C., December 13, 1972. Mimeographed.

———. Statement in U.S. Senate, Committee on Labor and Public Welfare, Subcommittee on Health, February 25, 1974. Mimeographed.

———. Statement in U.S. Senate, Select Committee on Small Business, Subcommittee on Monopoly, May 9, 1972. Mimeographed.

———. Statement in U.S. Senate, Select Committee on Small Business, Subcommittee on Monopoly, February 5, 1973. Mimeographed.

FDC Reports, "The Pink Sheet." See especially the following issues: December 4, 1972; July 2, 1973; April 1, 1974; August 16, 1974; September 16, 1974.

Finkel, Marion. "Investigational Drug Studies: Recent FDA Efforts." Speech before the Symposium on Clinical Pharmacological Methods, Phase 1-11, New Orleans, March 23, 1973. Mimeographed.

———. *Report on Use of Advisory Committees in Drug Regulation.* March 5, 1973. Mimeographed.

Hutt, Peter. "Safety Regulation in the Real World." Washington, D.C.:

National Academy of Sciences, May 15, 1973. Mimeographed.

Kennedy, Edward. "[Keynote] Address." Press release of speech before the Tulane Medical Symposium on Principles and Techniques of Human Research and Therapeutics, New Orleans, November 2, 1975. Mimeographed.

Rutstein, David P. Statement in U.S. Senate, Select Committee on Small Business, Subcommittee on Monopoly, February 6, 1973. Mimeographed.

Schmidt, Alexander. *The Commissioner's Report of Investigation of Charges.* October 24, 1975. Mimeographed.

———. "Communication as the Basis of Regulation." Food and Drug Law Institute/FDA, December 11, 1973. Mimeographed.

———. "Dimensions of Change in the FDA." Speech before the Pharmaceutical Advertising Seminar, Chicago, September 3, 1973. Mimeographed.

———. "The FDA Today: Critics, Congress, and Consumerism." Speech before the National Press Club, Washington, D.C., October 29, 1974.

———. "The FDA in 1985." Speech before the Tulane Medical Symposium on Principles and Techniques of Human Research and Therapeutics, New Orleans, November 5, 1975. Mimeographed.

———. Statement in U.S. Senate, Judiciary Committee, Subcommittee on Separation of Powers, July 21, 1975. Mimeographed.

———. Statement in U.S. Senate, Committee on Labor and Public Welfare, Subcommittee on Health, August 16, 1974. Mimeographed.

[Schultz, Harold.] "Risk-Benefit Considerations in Food Safety." Attachment A to minutes of November 14-15, 1974, joint meeting of National Advisory Food Committee and National Advisory Veterinary Medicine Committee, November 1974. Mimeographed.

Seidman, David. "Protection and Overprotection, the Politics and Economics of Pharmaceutical Regulation." Paper given at Midwest Political Science Association conference, April 29-May 1, 1976. Mimeographed.

Simmons, Henry. Statement in U.S. Senate, Select Committee on Small Business, Subcommittee on Monopoly, February 5, 1973. Also five addenda (A-E), and exhibits 4-18; and "Status Report on a Number of

Drugs Marketed Elsewhere but Not in This Country," later inserted for the record. Mimeographed.

Tishler, Max. *Reflections on Drug Research and Development.* Paper presented at a symposium at Churchill College, Cambridge, England, July 21-23, 1972. Mimeographed.

U.S. Department of Health, Education, and Welfare. Food and Drug Administration. *Annual Report,* 1974, preprint copy.

———. *FY 1976 PMS Blue Book.* April 1975. Mimeographed.

———. Listing of all hearings the Food and Drug Administration has participated in from 1973 to date. March 26, 1975. Mimeographed.

U.S. Department of Health, Education, and Welfare. Review Panel on New Drug Regulations. *Assessment of the Commissioner's Report of October 1975.* May 1976. Mimeographed.

U.S. Food and Drug Administration, National Advisory Drug Committee. *Summary Minutes.* April 20-21, 1972 (first meeting); September 28-29, 1972 (third meeting), with attached memorandum and with attached "Summary Statement" by the Committee; April 5, 1973 (fifth meeting); June 29, 1973 (sixth meeting); January 24-25, 1974 (eighth meeting); April 3-4, 1974 (ninth and last meeting), with attachments.

———. *Transcript* (official). September 28, 1972; September 29, 1972; June 29, 1973.

———. *Transcript* (unofficial). November 30, 1972, with mimeographed statements by Judge Aarons, Robert Dripps, Benjamin Gordon, Joseph Stetler, James Turner, Anita Johnson, and Sidney Wolfe.

———. *Transcript* (unofficial). December 1, 1972. Mimeographed.

U.S. Food and Drug Administration, National Advisory Food and Drug Committee. *Minutes.* March 27-28, 1975 (first meeting); June 24-25, 1975 (second meeting).

———. *Transcript* (official). November 20, 1975.

U.S. Senate, Select Committee on Small Business, Subcommittee on Monopoly. "Present Status of Competition in the Pharmaceutical Industry," transcript of testimony March 14, 1973; discussion includes Leonard Schriffin, Samuel Baker (separate statement), Sam Peltzman, and Stanley Lebergott. pp. 9988-10119. Mimeographed.

Wardell, William. *The Drug Lag: An International Comparison.* A preliminary draft, October 1972. Mimeographed.

———. *Introduction of New Therapeutic Drugs in the U.S. and Great Britain: An International Comparison.* A preliminary draft, November 1972. Mimeographed.

———. "Regulation of Drug Research and Therapeutic Practice." Statement in U.S. Senate, Select Committee on Small Business, Subcommittee on Health, September 27, 1974. Mimeographed.

———. "Regulation and Pharmaceutical Innovation: A Review of the Relationship Between Regulation Aimed at Protecting Health and Human Safety, and Innovation Leading to Medically Useful Drugs." Written for the National Science Foundation, June 1976. Mimeographed.